Feelin' Hot?

A Humorous, Informative and Truthful
Look at Menopause

Rebecca J. Hulem
RN, RNP, CNM
Certified Menopause
Clinician

Copyright 2003 by RJH Communications, LLC

All rights reserved.

No part of this book may be reproduced or utilized in any form or by any means, electronic or mechanical, including photocopying, recording or by any information storage and retrieval system without permission in writing.

Inquiries should be addressed to:

RJH Communications, LLC

5737 Kanan Road, #261

Agoura Hills, California 91301-1601

818-889-2475

First Edition

Library of Congress Cataloging-in-Publication Data:

Hulem, Rebecca J.

    Feelin' Hot? : *A Humorous, Informative and Truthful Look at Menopause*

    p.   cm.

    ISBN 0-9741618-0-2 (pbk.)

    1. Menopause 2. Women—Health

    3. Hormone therapy—Alternatives 4. Middle age—Women 5. Menopause— Social Aspects of

    2003094652   618.175 HU   RG 186 M48

Cover Illustration by: Jerri Conrado, JRC Promotions

Editor: Marianne Cotter

Printed in the United States of America

At Morgan Printing in Austin, Texas

This book is dedicated to my mother,
Elizabeth Jane Adams who unfortunately
did not live long enough to experience the
other side of menopause.

My daughter, Tracy Elizabeth Roemer who
I can only imagine with her tenacious spirit
will sail right through this phase of life.

And to all women who crave the
understanding to make informed choices
about their health through out mid-life.

Contents

Acknowledgements

Throughout my life I have been blessed with an extraordinary support system, one that is filled with family, friends, colleagues, and patients, almost all of whom have in some way encouraged me to write this book. My greatest support has been my husband and soul mate, Frederick Hulem. Thank you, my love, for the countless hours of editing, research, arranging, consulting and, of course, encouragement that kept me going whenever I entertained the thought of quitting. But most of all thank you for the acceptance and love that you continue to give me every day that we are together.

Gaining the courage to commit my voice to the written word required a considerable amount of coaxing. After all, who am I to think I might have something important to say that others will want to read? Just in the knick of time, the universe sent me two amazing women. I call them my guardian angels: Sylvia Acevedo and Janet Osimo. These two beautiful, amazing women took it upon themselves to fly out to California from Austin, Texas to conduct a focus group of seventeen enthusiastic women who were willing to help me find an answer to the question: What do women want to read on the subject of menopause? A big hug goes out to my sister, Julie Martin, and my dear friend, Patricia Caminiti, who rounded up all the women who attended the focus group that special evening in August of 2002. What a wonderful group of women who selflessly came together to support my dream. I have taken your candid feedback, suggestions, and comments to heart and, hopefully, have addressed your concerns regarding menopause.

Along the lines of candor I applaud my editor, Marianne Cotter, who contributed an endless supply of encouragement and insight with gentleness and patience, being very careful not to bruise my fragile beginning as a new writer. Her expertise and wisdom are reflected in every page of this book. Special acknowledgement also goes to Jerri Conrado from *JRC Promotions and Creative Strategies*, who not only designed the cover, but spent countless hours in the research and development of my business and in redesigning my website. I can only hope even a smidgen of her beauty, grace and style rubs off on me. When it comes to style I also have a big thank you for Toni Yamin of *Stylish Dressing by Toni*, who has dressed me to the nines with beautiful Don Castor clothing for my lecture tours.

Countless people in the medical field have contributed to my knowledge and expertise in women's health. First and foremost, my colleagues and peers at Kaiser Permanente where I spent twenty-five years perfecting my skills. I miss you all. To Dr. Linda Katz, Ob/Gyn extraordinaire, I thank you for always keeping a place for me in your office. And Elaine Blieden, pharmacist and consulting specialist on bio-identical compounding hormones for women, thank you for educating me and my patients on the benefits of bio-identical hormones. Most importantly, thank you for your continued support of my work and your valued friendship. Many thanks also to Dr. James Iwanoff, who taught me with his hands about the many healthful benefits of regular chiropractic adjustments. My neck, back and shoulders are grateful for every visit. A long hug goes to Karyn Maag-Weigand who, with gentleness and patience, led me to the life of my dreams. Thanks also to Sherrill Tillger, RN, MN-Director of

Professional Education Center, for giving me the jump-start that propelled me into the speaking business. Thank you Sherrill! I am deeply touched and very grateful for the continued support and encouragement of my work from Linzi Friedrich, Luna Brand Coordinator at Clif Bar Inc.

This list would not be complete without mentioning three very special people. First, my big sister Eloise Robertson who happens to think her little sister is very special. Second, my son Robert for his sweet and gentle nature and for adoring his lucky mother. No mother could ask for a more loving son. And finally, my very best friend Carol, whom I absolutely adore for her quick wit and tenacity in getting me safely to the top of every mountain we have climbed together. My soul beams whenever I am with you!

Introduction

Twenty seven years ago when I graduated from nursing school, it never occurred to me that some day I would be speaking and writing about the many wonderful aspects of transitioning through menopause. As a brand new nurse with the ideals of Florence Nightingale, my love was pregnant mothers and their babies. I had my career plan all mapped out. First I would work as a labor and delivery room nurse. Then, after I had mastered the skills in that area I would return to school and become an Ob/Gyn nurse practitioner. One of the wonderful aspects of having a nursing career is that you can continue your education in stages. And so I did, which became necessary as I found myself, like so many other women, in the position of being a single mother with two small children to support.

Fast-forward about twenty-two years and there I was, working as a certified nurse mid-wife (I went back to school more than once) for Kaiser Permanente, a very large health maintenance organization. In fact, up until January 2003 when I retired, most of my nursing practice and education was obtained through this wonderful organization. Kaiser, because of its large membership, also provided me the opportunity to meet and care for thousands of women transitioning through all stages of their life, from puberty through menopause.

It was when I was working as a nurse midwife in my mid-forties when the first signs of the mid-life change (perimenopause) descended on me. Physically, I felt like I had run into a brick wall. I had no energy or patience for the simplest everyday tasks. Even the drive to work was becoming a trial. Dealing with traffic and finding a parking space—all the annoying aspects of daily life that I had accepted long ago—were suddenly grating on my nerves, putting me in a bad mood. Too often I let my moods affect my interactions with my coworkers, and even, sadly, my patients.

I continued this moody existence for several months, thinking that everyone around me had become intollerable until one day a dear patient of mine, whose baby I had just delivered, gathered up her courage and confronted me. "Rebecca," she said. "You must have been having a bad day when you delivered my baby." "Why?" I asked, somewhat surprised at her remark. "Well, you snapped at me and raised your voice several times while giving me instructions during my last stage of labor. Never, in all the years that I have been coming to you for my health care, have you spoken to me like that."

I was devastated. We all have bad days and bad moods, but it's not my nature to treat anyone in such an unkind and unprofessional manner. Thanks to this courageous patient, I stopped and took an honest look at myself. I started paying careful attention to my moods, feelings, physical symptoms and behavior when interacting with other people. I realized that, in addition to becoming impatient, I also had become distracted. Plus I was having a very difficult time getting to sleep, and was suffering through migraine headaches every other week. But most discouraging was the realization that I had lost my passion for working with pregnant mothers and their babies, a passion I thought would carry me blissfully to the end of my nursing career.

So, just when we think we have life all figured out,

everything changes. It's normal to feel apprehensive about change, but if we open ourselves up to it, change can be a wonderful opportunity to explore our potential and grow in new ways.

And this is how I have come to feel about a phase in our life called menopause. Yes, menopause is a powerful physical transition that we must all endure. And yes, it can also be confusing not knowing whether you are in full-blown menopause or in the preliminary perimenopause stage.

The recent findings from the Women's Health Initiative Study have confused the issue even more. How do you successfully treat the bothersome symptoms of menopause without putting yourself at greater risk for life-robbing situations like breast cancer, uterine cancer, heart attack, stroke, blood clots and dementia?

The choices are mind-boggling. Do you start on a course of conventional hormone replacement therapy? If so, how long do you use it before putting yourself at greater risk for life-threatening situations? Or do you take less conventional approaches like bio-identical compounding hormones? Or do you skip hormones altogether and enter the world of herbs and dietary supplements?

But the worst problem for most women is that they just don't have the knowledge, the understanding or the time to reach informed decisions with which they are comfortable. And, too often the medical community falls short of providing the support you need to make the best choices for you. Many doctors simply tell you the facts as they know them and then expect you to make a quick decision.

So, is it reasonable to say that all this confusion has you *Feelin' Hot?* I'm not just talking about the hot flashes that wake you up at night in a sweat. I'm talking figuratively about sweating out the very important decisions you have to make with very little direction. You simply don't have the understanding and knowledge to respond to the hard questions you are facing.

If this is the case, *Feelin' Hot?* will give you a simple, yet powerful basis to begin sorting out the confusion. I have taken many steps, both personal and professional, to prepare myself for the writing of this book.

- First and foremost, I identified and addressed my own menopausal symptoms and sought out the solutions that best suited my personal health history.
- Secondly, through the many private and public seminars I have taught over the years, I have helped hundreds of women identify which areas of their health histories to focus on while transitioning through this complex phase in their lives.
- In addition, I have treated hundreds of women as patients during my career with Kaiser Permanente and, recently, in my own private practice, women who are experiencing symptoms caused by the perimenopause and menopause transition.
- And, as a final preparation, I held a focus group to find out what women really want to read about menopause. I listened to many wonderful women share their stories, their frustrations and their hopes for a

better understanding of what is happening in their bodies. I listened to their uncertainty as to how to move forward. After all, menopause signals a change, not an end. It is the signpost of a new beginning into the second half of life.

The women who participated in the focus group, which was held in August 2002, were in all phases of perimenopause and menopause. Their moods during the several hours we spent together went from light-hearted to serious and contemplative. The following is a synopsis of the most important points they made.

- The tone of the book was very important. Humor, respect, a positive attitude and hope were all viewed as desired attributes. You will find the chapter titles to be humorous and light-hearted, with relevant content and down-to-earth suggestions on how to manage many of the menopause symptoms discussed.
- Topics included in a book on menopause must cover a wide range of issues, including biological and physiological explanations, symptoms (mood swings, hot flashes, memory and sleep disturbances, decreased libido, weight changes), complications (osteoporosis) and lifestyle choices (nutrition, diet, exercise). And the very controversial issue of hormone replacement therapy must be addressed. Surprisingly though, information regarding heart disease did not come up. But as you will read in this book, heart disease is the number one killer of women over the age of 50. You will find out why this is so when you read Chapter 8, *"Let's Get to the Heart of the Matter."*

- When discussing the controversial issues around prescribing hormone replacement therapy, many participants felt that their doctors were all too eager to prescribe hormones or other medications without asking questions and without consideration of the woman's unique needs. And, if options were discussed, the women in the focus group felt that their own preferences were not taken into consideration.

- When I held a vote by secret ballot to get their reaction to titles of existing books, the number one favorite was *"Screaming to be Heard: Hormonal Connections Women Suspect and Doctors Still Ignore"* by Elizabeth Lee Vilet M.D. Most women picked this one because they identified strongly with the words "screaming to be heard," which reflected their frustration at not being taken seriously, listened to or understood by their physicians or their families. Many women expressed feelings of isolation and felt that they were on their own to figure out how to best treat their menopause symptoms.

- Last but never least, was the issue of decreased libido. Many women expressed huge disappointment that they were no longer as interested in sex as they once were. The women in the focus group were in many different stages of relationships with their partners, from newlyweds to being married for 30 years, to recently dating. But one concern shared by almost all the women in the group was that the men in their lives felt responsible for the woman's lack of sexual interest. The women felt very strongly that a chapter dealing with the effects of menopause on libido should be included in the book and that it should be interesting enough for men to want to read as well.

Relying on my personal and professional experience along with input from the focus group, I went to work on this book, *Feelin' Hot?* I always kept my focus on you, the reader.

Each chapter has a major theme, which relates to the multitude of symptoms that most women experience while transitioning through this wonderful stage of life. You will find that the defining message of this book is carried out on almost every page. What is that message? **Many women, many choices.**

The last chapter of this book is called, What's a Woman to Do? There I introduce a revolutionary method I have designed to help you make decisions about managing your menopausal symptoms and maintaining a lifetime of health. It is called the S.H.O.P method, and it is based on a shopping metaphor. Every woman loves to SHOP, but no woman likes to be SOLD! I will give you tools to use that will end the confusion when shopping for long-term health.

Follow me now as we start with Chapter One: In the beginning, *My Mother, My Self.*
Enjoy....

Chapter 1

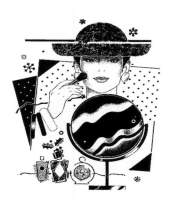

My Mother, Myself

The journey in between what you once were and who you are now becoming is where the dance of life really takes place.
— *Barbara De Angelis,*
Inspiration About Love

I'm not my mother.
I'm not my mother.
I'm not my mother!
Oh My God, I'm becoming my mother!

Do you remember how you felt when you first noticed the changes in your mother's body and behavior? I recall being worried.

"What's happening to her?" I wondered. "She's a bit out of control with her eating. She's getting bigger around the waist and her stomach is sticking out in a really unattractive way. She buys pants with elastic waistbands and her underwear is from Fruit of the Loom. Hmm…whatever happened to those sexy little numbers she used to order from the Spiegel catalog?" And, I have noticed, she can't remember anything. I tell her important things that are happening in my life, and the next day she doesn't remember a thing I said. I hate to sound critical, but mom is losing it."

Guess what? If you are reading this book, the person being described above is not your mother. You may not be ready for the "M" word yet, but get ready for a wild ride because it's your turn now.

In The Beginning - Biology Basics

While hormones may be the culprits instigating these seemingly sudden changes in your body, age is the catalyst. Mid-life changes in a woman's body can start as early as the late 30s. However, most women don't become aware of the changes until they reach their 40s. In high school biology you learned that your ovaries had millions of tiny follicles that would someday be transformed into eggs. Well, about those eggs...

Is Your Egg Basket Empty?

You are now somewhere in mid-life, probably in your 40s, and the egg basket—your ovaries—have very few, if any, viable eggs. When, and if, your ovaries produce a golden egg every month, they also produce three very lively hormones that can be characterized as two wise women and a male tag-a-long. They are, of course, estrogen, progesterone and our male friend, testosterone.

Estrogen and progesterone are the two wise female hormones that work together to make you the amazing woman you are. Estrogen, which is produced by your ovaries, adrenal glands and fat cells, can be thought of as the goddess of hormones, because she oversees, to a great extent, the well-being of your brain, bones, skin, breast, heart, uterus and vagina.

Feelin' Hot?

Unlike estrogen, progesterone is produced solely by the ovaries and then only when ovulation occurs. While progesterone keeps you and your body functioning in many small ways, its main job is to regulate menstrual periods and support a pregnancy in its early stages until the placenta can take over.

Lastly, testosterone—that male tag-a-long—also performs several jobs. However, his main one is to provide you with the sex drive—that desire to have sex. He is produced by your ovaries and adrenal glands in equal amounts.

This wonderful process of hormone production winds down as you age. Ovulation no longer occurs as it once did, resulting in a progression of changes in your body and your mind.

Welcome to Mid-life! An Equal Opportunity Experience for Women Everywhere

The first sign of your life change may be that your menstrual periods refuse to adhere to their usual schedule. Women come into my office every day complaining that their cycles are changing. "They always come every 28 days." "I've never missed a period in my life (except when I was pregnant), but it didn't come last month." "My periods are lasting longer." "My periods are shorter." "I have more cramps than usual." "Give me a quick fix so I can go on with my life." Sound familiar? As women, we have always reserved the right to complain about the inconveniences of our periods. But did you ever think you would complain that your period has a mind of its own, or that you miss it or worry about it when it becomes less reliable? Always and never are dead end streets.

If you are in your late 30s or early 40s, change becomes the operative word. Let's discover what's really happening.

Perimenopause: Change Means You Are Still Alive

When a woman frantically tells me that her periods are changing, I always think "transition." The medical industry calls this time in a woman's life perimenopause. Perimenopause is the beginning of a major physical, emotional, and psychological change in your life, and it is just as powerful as the one you went through when you started puberty.

Perimenopause, which literally means "around the menopause," is an indication that you're almost there (menopause), but you still have some time left. But before you get to menopause you will probably experience changes in your body and mind that you never dreamed possible.

Let's take your moods as an example. Your moods may become so erratic they can be measured on the Richter scale. And when mood swings are set in motion, patience is no longer one of your virtues.

You may also find that the abundance of energy that once helped you balance your responsibilities has disappeared into thin air. And memory, that wonderful faculty that helped you to know where you put your car keys, sun glasses and your best friend's name, may now elude you when you most need it. And of course, the picture would not be complete without the occasional hot flash. "Why do I need hot flashes?" you may ask. Well, because without the occasional hot flash, especially at night, you would be sleeping soundly. That's right. Changes in sleep patterns may also show up at this wonderful stage of life. "I can't deal with this. Not now, I'm too busy," you say.

Feelin' Hot?

What Can I Do?

When I was writing this book, my husband said I should tell my readers that "nothing can be done" to make it any easier. After all, he lived with me throughout this phase in my life.

But he's not entirely correct. Many options are available to help ease your passage through this transition. For example, I mentioned earlier that hormones cause changes in your body. One of these hormones, progesterone, is the major cause of most perimenopausal symptoms, since it is responsible for the critical task of regulating your periods. It also balances your moods, gets you to sleep at night, and provides the energy necessary to keep up with your hectic life. As I said earlier, this hormone is only produced when ovulation occurs and since ovulation is no longer occurring on a regular, predictable schedule, the production of progesterone, to which your body has become accustomed, is now dropping. So the key to easing the symptoms of perimenopause is to replace the progesterone that your ovaries are no longer producing.

There Are Choices!

Today, there are many choices. Of course, you will start by visiting your doctor or health care practitioner who will carefully evaluate your individual medical history before advising any course of action. Your doctor will discuss several choices with you, including:

- Progesterone by prescription, either in a synthetic or bio-identical compounded form. Your health care practitioner should explain all the dosage issues, including length of time each month that you take the medication. He or she should also explain the difference between a synthetic or bio-identical compounded form of progesterone.

Which one is better? The best answer is the one that reduces your symptoms, and causes the least side affects. In my professional experience, micronized progesterone or bio-identical compounded progesterone appears to cause the least side effects. Micronized is a fancy name that means small particle size. The trade name for the commercially produced, micronized progesterone is Prometrium.

- Low dose birth control pills. Birth control pills now come in much lower dosages than when they first became available. And, they can be safely prescribed to women over the age of 35. But to take birth control pills safely you must be a non-smoker with blood pressure and cholesterol levels within normal ranges. The use of birth control pills during the perimenopause transition will regulate your irregular periods, provide solid protection against a surprise pregnancy, and relieve most of the symptoms described earlier.

- Intrauterine Device (IUD). If you are having heavy, long periods and need birth control as well, a new IUD called the Mirena is now on the market. With this method, over time, your periods may become very light or almost non-existent. It will also protect you from an unwanted pregnancy. Remember, your ovaries cannot be completely trusted at this time in your life.

Feelin' Hot?

You may still have one more egg in the ovary basket just waiting to be hatched!

Do I Have To Take Drugs?

You might be asking yourself, "Do I have to take prescription drugs?" Well, the answer is "No, not at all." These are just a few options that are available to women who really need them.

There are a variety of more natural options, including progesterone creams that can be bought over the counter at most health food stores. Some women have found these creams to be helpful in relieving their symptoms. Others have found no relief at all. Just knowing that there are a variety of options available reassures most women. Remember, your mother didn't have these options. She probably suffered in silence. But don't beat yourself up for criticizing your mother. We all did. Besides, she's your mother. She will always forgive you.

Menopause – Am I There Yet?

Now, let's move on to the next phase of mid-life: menopause. But before we do, let me answer one question that comes up with almost every patient I see. "How do I know if I'm in perimenopause or menopause?" The answer to that question is really very simple. You are in perimenopause if you are still having periods of any kind; long, short, heavy, or light, with or without cramps. Until you have gone one full year without any bleeding or spotting, you are still in perimenopause.

This brings me now to the formal definition of menopause:

Menopause is the end of menstruation and, therefore, the end of your childbearing years.

The average age of menopause is 51. Yes, you can go through it at an earlier age, and yes, you can go through it at a later age. But most of us will experience it in our early 50s. Some women may have had a hysterectomy, but still have their ovaries intact. If this is your situation, you will still experience perimenopause and menopausal symptoms. You just won't have a menstrual period to gauge which "phase" of mid-life you are in.

The symptoms that occur in mid-life can make you feel crazy enough. But when you don't even know which phase you're in or what to call it, you can really feel crazy.

This was my situation. I had a hysterectomy in my early 40s and still had my ovaries intact. I was breezing along, actually enjoying not having a period, when all of a sudden, without warning, I started to experience extreme fatigue, mood swings and sleepless nights. I had no idea what was going on. Given my 20-year career working in women's health, you would think that I would have recognized these perimenopausal symptoms.

I was clueless.

I thought my mood swings were the result of my colleagues' and coworkers' incompetence. I actually thought that if I could just get my coworkers to work by my rules, I wouldn't be so moody. I thought my fatigue was a result of working long hours. Boy was I surprised to later find out that all these symptoms were a result of being in perimenopause. Needless to say, I had to make a lot of apologies to my coworkers, husband and children for my "strange behavior." If this sounds familiar, take comfort in knowing you are not experiencing this new phase of life alone. Approximately 40 million American women are going through this transition at the same time you are. Around the globe we are 470 million women strong. And what a wonderful group we are.

Beginnings and Endings

Menopause is the poetry of beginnings and endings. It is the end of worrying about menstrual periods and the right choice of birth control. It is the beginning of a new phase. This new phase is one in which you can now act on the dreams you have harbored over the years; the things you always said you would do when you had time; dreams of starting your own business, writing a bestselling book, traveling around the world, or raising money for your favorite cause. We all have these dreams. The question is will you give yourself permission to address them now? But wait, you say, "Isn't there a little bit more to menopause than no more periods?" Well, yes there is.

Riding on the Symptom Express

The full menopause stage sees an increase in perimenopausal symptoms. Hot flashes may become more intense and more frequent. Regulating body temperature is just one of the many jobs that estrogen performs in your body. A drop in estrogen levels causes hot flashes when your menstrual periods no longer occur. Or, if you have had a hysterectomy and still have your ovaries, hot flashes will start to occur when your ovaries run out of eggs.

Hot flashes happen suddenly, without warning, and often at the most in opportune moments: in the middle of a very important meeting with your boss, or while explaining to your 16-year-old why he or she cannot use the family car.

Hot flashes typically occur at night, sometimes all night, especially at two in the morning. Every woman's body is different, of course, but most women don't escape this phase without at least one hot flash. If you are not sure whether or not you've had one, you haven't. Like knowing that you've had a true labor contraction or an orgasm, there is no doubt in your mind when the real thing comes along.

In addition to hot flashes and night sweats, you may also experience the following: itchy skin, achy joints and more short-term memory loss. More short-term memory loss, you ask? Keep in mind that this is a time of tremendous fluctuation in your ovarian hormones. With fluctuation in hormones, you will experience physical and emotional changes until your body adjusts. Many of these symptoms will fade away as your body regains its balance. And be assured, your body will regain its balance. How long the entire process will take in your body cannot be predicted. On average, it takes two to five years. Now don't fret, you won't be bothered with symptoms every day. There will be some days that you won't even know that you are in menopause.

This brings me to another question. Have you noticed lately that your children (young or old) are jumping in to help you complete your sentences? Our children can become very impatient with us when we just can't find the right word to say what we mean.

Memory Loss: Who Took My Car?

There is also the issue of disorientation. Picture this: you leaving the mall after a wonderful day of shopping the sales. You are so proud of yourself. With coupons, you bought that darling top, which was originally priced at $39.99, for just $5.02. Wow! Can life feel any better? You go out to the parking lot, and walk down the aisle toward your car. Now you are standing in the exact spot where your car should be parked and, wouldn't you know, someone moved it! You panic at first. Then you slowly look around, hoping no one is watching, and realize that, in your excitement, you walked out the wrong door of the department store! You decide to keep this one a secret. No one needs to know.

And The Symptoms Keep On Coming

Add to the scenario above a few more symptoms, and a truly frustrating time of life emerges. You may, from time to time, experience a spontaneous loss of urine when you cough, sneeze, laugh, or run. Add to that vaginal dryness, that sandpapery, dried up feeling that makes you feel like sex is impossible. Loss of urine and vaginal dryness usually occur when your estrogen levels are at their lowest. Among the many services estrogen (the goddess of all hormones) performs, are lubricating the vagina and supporting the muscles in the vagina that surround the opening to the bladder.

And let's add one last symptom to the list: decreased libido—otherwise known as the realization that you have no interest or desire to have sex, ever again. It's like cooking. You've been cooking and enjoying it for 30 years and suddenly you have absolutely no desire to cook even your favorite dishes.

Where's That Light at The End of The Tunnel?

I know. I know. You're probably wondering if there is anything that could possibly fix all these symptoms. Well, actually there is. No woman should have to walk around having hot flashes, mood swings, sleep disturbances, disorientation, leaky bladders, and absolutely no interest in sex.

Let's go back to the three very important hormones that

are produced by the ovaries: estrogen, progesterone and that male tag-a-long, testosterone. In perimenopause, it is the progesterone that is on the low side and out of balance with estrogen. In menopause you now have very little, if any, progesterone and estrogen, and your testosterone may be on the low side as well.

Why is estrogen so important? As I mentioned earlier, estrogen affects almost every organ in a woman's body. Your brain, breasts, skin, bones, uterus, and vagina all need some level of estrogen to stay in good working order. How much is needed varies from woman to woman. Testosterone, even though it is predominantly a male hormone, is also produced in a woman's body. Testosterone has been called the hormone of desire. Those fantasies you may have once had about your favorite actor were brought to you by none other than the hormone, testosterone. This hormone is also important for muscle strength and, to some degree, strong bones.

Hormone Replacement?

Now you know that many of the major symptoms during menopause are the result of declining ovarian hormones. So, you would think the easiest solution would be to replace these hormones and be on your way. Not so fast! You may have heard a lot of commotion lately regarding the benefits and risks of hormone replacement therapy.

The Women's Health Initiative, a large clinical trial involving two very common hormones that have been used for years to help ease the symptoms of menopause, released its study results in July 2002. The two hormones are Premarin and Provera. Premarin is an estrogen product and Provera is a progestin. The trade name for these products when combined in one pill is called PremPro. These hormones are

Feelin' Hot?

given together either in one pill or two separate pills to women who are having bothersome menopausal symptoms.

Preliminary research also suggested that Premarin and Provera would help protect a woman from developing heart disease, which is the number one killer of women over 50. So, the Women's Health Initiative set out to prove that in addition to relieving the bothersome symptoms of menopause, PremPro would also protect women from heart disease. What the study actually found was just the opposite. They determined that some of the women who were taking Prempro actually had more heart attacks, strokes and invasive breast cancer.

There is still much debate within the medical and research communities over the validity of the study. But, debate or no debate, the study results and the subsequent media coverage has caused fear and confusion for women all over the world. The medical community has also been impacted in terms of what to tell patients. Should women taking hormones stop? Should women who are considering hormones look for alternative treatments? Since the study only covered two of the many hormones available, is it fair to assume that all hormones are dangerous?

I'm sure you can see the huge dilemma here. And since you are reading this book, you probably feel the confusion as well. No one has all the answers yet. There is still much research to be done, leaving medical professionals and women alike with more questions than answers. But, if you get nothing else from this book, please get this: You are a unique and important woman. You deserve the best from your health care provider. Make sure he or she gives you the time and attention necessary to answer your questions thoroughly.

You Are Unique

The most useful result of The Women's Health Initiative study so far is the understanding that there are many women and, there are many choices! There is no one dosage or method of treatment that is appropriate for all menopausal women. There is no blanket time frame during which women should take hormones. Each and every woman should be evaluated according to her individual medical history. The many variables of your unique history will determine if hormones are the right choice for you.

In the chapters that follow, we will take an in-depth look at each symptom mentioned in this chapter along with tips on how to best manage each of them. When we get to Chapter 5, *"Stuck in Hormone Hell,"* we'll deal with hormones in great detail.

By the way, the symptoms that appear during mid-life get a lot of attention. They can be hard to ignore. But your heart and bones are the most important players when it comes to your long-term health. Let me show you how…

Chapter 2

Perimenopause
Also Known as... Where Did I Put My Keys?

> **Happiness is good health and a bad memory**
> **— Ingrid Bergman**

"What's happening to me?"

This is the question I hear most often from women going through mid-life. And it goes on from there: "I can't remember a thing. I've never had to make a list or carry a daily planner before. Now, not only do I need them, I can't remember where I put them."

You are not alone. When I sat down to write this chapter, I couldn't for the life of me remember a thing I wanted to say. Even with an outline, nothing was coming to me. I panicked. Does this sound familiar?

Memory, that wonderful ability to recall names, words, where you put things, and what to do next, often starts to fade during the perimenopause stage of life. Frustrating experiences like losing your car keys and forgetting where you parked your car become daily occurrences. You may feel so distracted that you can't remember why you walked into a room or whose number you just dialed on the phone. Your children complain that you are not listening to them. You may even forget that you have children!

At some point after your 30s and before menopause, you will notice that you have become forgetful. Keeping simple things straight becomes harder and harder as your hormones start to fluctuate.

It's difficult to isolate the cause of female mid-life memory problems because so many complex changes are taking place in your body during this time. I will, however, discuss some of the current theories.

Estrogen and Receptor Sites

Much of the blame for mid-life forgetfulness is attributed to estrogen, one of the "two wise women" hormones. Actually, estrogen is responsible for almost all of the uncomfortable symptoms associated with menopause. While our knowledge of estrogen is not complete, we do know that estrogen receptor sites (areas in your body that are begging for a visit from estrogen) exist in just about every major organ, including the brain. Being the body's most complex organ, the brain is particularly sensitive to changes in estrogen levels. So, if you ever feel that you're literally losing your mind, just blame it on fluctuating estrogen levels.

Why is estrogen so important to the brain? When estrogen travels to the brains' receptor sites, it helps activate processes that stimulate the brain to think and remember. Estrogen also helps the brain retrieve glucose from our blood stream, which is used as fuel. Without the help of glucose, thinking processes would slow down. In this way, estrogen levels can affect memory, learning, mood and attention span. Fortunately, the ovaries don't carry the sole burden of producing estrogen. Because so many of our organs need it to function properly, estrogen is produced in many ways by our bodies. Among the organs and processes that produce estrogen are the adrenal glands and a conversion process from fat cells.

Our Brains, Our Gender

Although it is probably futile to go in this direction, many women ask if men have similar problems with memory loss at mid-life.

Men have their forgetful moments too, but they don't have as many things on their plate to remember as we do. We are responsible for so much in terms of taking care of others that we are more aware of and troubled by memory problems than men.

We've always known that our brains process information differently than men's. What you may not know (or perhaps have forgotten) is that men are more factually oriented than women. Their brains focus on the bottom line; remembering facts, dates and times, usually as applied to their work.

We women, however, are more relationship oriented, and maintaining the quality of our relationships is very important to us. Forgetting someone's name or not being able to articulate thoughts and feelings is very disturbing to a woman.

It also seems that men are more willing than women to use props, especially technology tools, to boost their memories. For men, the more technology tools the better—maybe it's that XY chromosome thing. My husband, for example, has a Palm Pilot that he has programmed with his important telephone numbers, addresses, work schedule and meetings—all the details that keep his life together. And, as if that's not enough, he also has a specialized cell phone that he programs to beep throughout the day with important reminders. This approach drives me crazy. I have neither the time nor the patience to program these gadgets and neither do most of the women I talk to. We generally use cell phones to connect with other people and when we can't remember whose number we just dialed, we are saved when the person's name is displayed on the screen. For women, this is the perfect use of a technology tool.

But we might be able to learn something from how men cope. They generally don't over-analyze or fret over memory lapses. They acknowledge that they could use some help, and then they go out and find the best tool for the job. Hmm…too bad this doesn't work with the perfect piece of jewelry.

Accepting Change

You now know that when you reach your 40s or 50s, you may experience difficulty in recalling things that once came easily. As a woman, you take pride in doing everything well and, no doubt; you want to continue functioning at the same high level. But don't be hard on yourself. Take a deep breath and realize that your world—and all the people in it—won't fall apart if you are not hyper-efficient 24-hours a day. The pressure will ease; improving your ability to stay on top of things and helping you remember to pick up your kids from school.

Acceptance is the first step to peace of mind. Yes, life changes and so does your body. Then be open to trying new approaches. Insanity has been defined as doing the same thing over and over and expecting different results. If you've reached a point in your life where you can't remember everything you have to do without making a list, then perhaps it is time to

Feelin' Hot?

start making lists.

You are not alone in this process. Take comfort in knowing that you are a member of a community of millions of women who are dealing with the same internal challenges. Know, too, that some days will be better than others in the memory department. When I teach seminars for women who are going through menopause, there are days when I am right on target—my thoughts flow into words effortlessly, and I sail through my presentation without skipping a beat. Other days, I can't think of the words to save my soul. So I let myself off the hook by giving permission to the women in front to finish my sentences for me. They love it, especially when they can think of the word and I can't.

The next step is to explore the many choices available to help you deal with the symptoms. The choices you make may be quite different from the ones your best friend makes. This is fine. You may also need to try several different approaches before you find the one that works best for you. Patience is a virtue at this time of life, patience to allow things to work.

A Balanced Program

Enjoying health and well being during this time of your life is achieved through a balanced program. Let's consider the following areas:

1. Nutrition
2. Exercise
3. Vitamin supplements and
4. Possible hormone replacement

Proper nutrition and exercise, in my opinion, are the two

must-haves in any mid-life program. Proper nourishment, accomplished by healthy eating habits, will feed every cell in your body. A healthy cell is a happy cell and a happy cell stays healthy. It's that simple.

Nutrition – The Key to Good Health

Nutrition is a very complex subject; so complex, in fact, that most professors in medical school don't even approach the subject. As a result, your physician is unlikely to address your eating habits and nutritional needs at this time in your life.

If you are a mother, you have, no doubt, made a point of learning enough about nutrition to instill good eating habits in your children. But what constitutes a good nutritional program at this transitional stage of your life? Simply put, you can never eat too many fruits, vegetables, and whole grains. These three food sources provide the majority of the vitamins, minerals and energy that your body needs each day to run at peak performance. You need small amounts of plant-based protein as well.

Unfortunately, most of us are too busy juggling multiple responsibilities to plan daily meals that include a wide variety of fruits and vegetables. The good news is that it is never too late to change your eating habits. As you age and realize that your body doesn't bounce back from neglect as quickly as it once did, you are more motivated to give it the nutrients it craves. As I will remind you many times in this book, your body is an amazing entity, resilient and forgiving. Once you experience improved memory and energy levels from proper nutrition, you will never go back to burgers and fries.

As you know, countless books and articles expound on the benefits of a high protein, low carbohydrate diet. In my

Feelin' Hot?

opinion, the problem with any food plan that excludes a food group is that it will also exclude nutrients that your body needs as it ages.

If you are concerned about your weight and still want to pursue good nutrition, an excellent book that covers both topics is: *Out Smarting the Mid-life Fat Cell* by Debra Waterhouse, M.P.H., R.D. If weight is your concern, read it for its excellent step-by-step balanced process of weight loss. Or, read it for its sound advice on good nutritional eating. It covers all the bases.

Exercise – The Path to a Healthier Life

Why take up exercise at mid-life? Excellent reasons include:

- Improved circulation throughout the body, bringing higher levels of oxygen to the brain. Your brain relies on oxygen to feed each cell.
- Increased serotonin levels in the brain, which help even out mood changes.
- Stress reduction. Although stress is always present, women handle it differently than men. As a woman, we fret, worry, analyze and attach ourselves to our stress. In other words, we internalize and become one with the stressful situation. Men, on the other hand, separate themselves from stress. They feel the stress, but then look for a solution. They do not generally take ownership of the stress. As a woman you need to exercise to reduce the toll that stress takes on your body, while helping you burn calories.
- If exercise is not part of your daily routine, and you could use some encouragement, check out Chapter 7,

"*Weight No More.*" There, I will talk about the kinds of exercise that best benefit your body and mind at this time of life. I also suggest ways to get started and stay motivated to continue.

Hormone Replacement—A Possible Key to Symptom Relief

Hormone replacement is another choice to explore. I will be talking about hormones, their benefits and risks in detail in Chapter 5, "*Stuck in Hormone Hell.*" For now, suffice it to say that some women experience positive benefits from hormones, including improved moods, a good night's sleep, and fewer and/or less intense hot flashes. It stands to reason that if you are getting adequate sleep and have fewer hot flashes to deal with, your moods will be better, reducing stress and increasing your capacity to cope with your myriad responsibilities. When you feel in better control of your life, your memory will be sharper as well. The science of whether or not hormones help improve memory is still evolving with many studies in progress.

Alternative Choices—Exploring Holistic Approaches

Some women don't want to take hormones or are advised against it by their physicians due to previous health issues. The beauty of this time of life is that there are almost as many choices as there are women. A holistic approach to mid-life symptoms is a preference for many women. What do we mean by holistic? Generally, a holistic approach focuses on the "whole" person—mind, body and spirit—rather than on the body's individual parts.

Feelin' Hot?

Many women are exploring alternatives to hormones such as botanicals, herbs and vitamin supplements. Unlike hormones, which require a prescription, these so-called "natural" substances can be bought over the counter. These more natural approaches may seem safer at first, but, since they are not regulated or monitored by the FDA, their safety and efficacy has not been established. For this reason, most health care professionals have concerns about their use.

What's the safest way to approach botanicals, herbs and vitamin supplements? Find a practitioner—a naturopathic physician—who specializes in advising women on these products. A naturopathic physician knows how these products work and which ones are best for you. Many herbal remedies are advertised for relief of menopause symptoms. These remedies combine several different herbs into one product. Combining herbs safely requires specialized training, which a naturopathic physician has. Just because herbs are derived from plant sources and are considered natural, doesn't mean that they aren't powerful.

If you would like to read more on this subject, the best book that I have come across is: *Female and Forgetful*, by Elisa Lottor, Ph.D., N.D. and Nancy P. Bruning. This book takes you through a six-step program to restore your memory and sharpen your mind. This book supports a sound nutritional program, regular exercise and discusses supplementation with herbal products, along with the scientific research to back it up.

Too Many Choices?

You may find all these choices confusing. If you're wondering how to make the best choice for you, let me give you a preview of coming attractions. In the last chapter of this book I will introduce you to the SHOP method, a revolutionary new program that I designed to help women sort through the choices available for relieving menopause symptoms. No more guessing, no more fretting. By following this step-by-step method you will effortlessly come to the decision best suited to you. As preparation, here are three words to focus on whenever you are faced with a decision about what "you" should do:

- Belief
- Preference
- Intuition

The Power of Your Beliefs

By including belief, preference and intuition in your decision-making process, you will be better able to navigate the options available to manage your menopause symptoms. Many women leave the decision-making process to their health care practitioners without considering their own instincts.

Let's say you are trying to decide between hormones and herbs to improve your memory during menopause. What is your belief about hormones? Do you believe they are safe? Do you believe that they will help you? What are your beliefs about herbs? Do you believe they will work as well and with fewer side effects than hormones? You have your own beliefs about hormones and herbal medications, but you have probably never been encouraged to take them seriously before. Your beliefs are powerful.

Every well-designed study of a medication includes a placebo group. Placebo refers to an inactive substance used as a control in an experiment. The people in the placebo group don't know that they aren't taking the real medication. But this group often reports positive results, anyway. Why? Because they believed that the medication they received was the real thing and would work as it was designed to. Becoming aware of your beliefs and honoring them will put power behind your decision every time.

Respect Your Preferences and Intuition

What are your preferences? Do you prefer to take hormones or do you prefer to take herbs? What is your intuition telling you to do? Intuition, as defined by Webster, is: "The act or faculty of knowing without the use of rational processes; immediate cognition." As I discussed earlier, our brain structure gives us women superior access to our intuition. Intuition is truly a woman's best friend.

How can intuition help us manage our menopause symptoms in mid-life? Now, more than any other time in our lives, we need to pay close attention to our feelings and hunches. These gut feelings come from an inner knowledge that guides us in the right direction. Whenever you find yourself in a quandary, stop, breathe in and out slowly, and allow your feelings to talk to you. This is your intuition speaking. If you take the time to listen to your intuition, you will make the decision that is right for you. Your health care provider can educate you as to the differences, benefits and the risks of your options, but the final decision is yours alone.

There's no need to feel locked into your choices. If you find that the hormones or herbs you decided to try are failing to meet your expectations, just make a switch. It's that simple. Remember, one size, one approach, does not work for all women.

Now, let's move on to the next chapter and take a look at how to get a good night's sleep.

Chapter 3

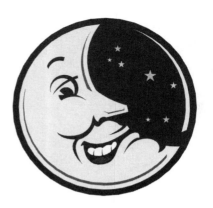

While You Are Not Sleeping

> *To dream the impossible,*
> *first you must sleep.*
> *— Marianne Cotter*

If you are like most women, mid-life marks the first time since you married and started a family that you can enjoy being alone. The kids have left the nest, bringing to an end the day-to-day responsibilities of parenthood. You have earned the right to relax and get a good night's sleep. No more waiting up, long past curfew, worrying about where your teenagers are. You and your partner have waited eagerly for this moment. Ah, alone at last.

The house is quiet. There are no distractions. Tomorrow is a busy day and you're looking forward to a good night's sleep, seven or eight hours of uninterrupted bliss. You plan to drift effortlessly into a deep, dreamy state. At least that was your plan.

Welcome to Reality

So you go through your usual nightly routine, taking off your makeup, cleansing and moisturizing your face. You apply the anti-aging cream (on which you just spent a fortune) in all the strategic places. No more sagging, no more wrinkles. It says so right on the jar. You may have to wait 6 to 12 weeks to see the results, but that's OK, you've got time. After brushing and flossing your teeth you take one last look at yourself in the mirror. You find that you're pleased at the woman staring back at you, even if you don't have your glasses on. Now you settle into your inviting bed, adjusting the pillows, getting cozy and warm under the covers. "Come, Mr. Sandman," you think, "I'm ready for you."

But he doesn't come. You change positions. You check the clock. It's already 11:30 p.m. But that's OK. If you fall asleep soon you will still get six hours of sleep. If you have a male partner, he is probably snoring already. But you're feeling anxious. "What's wrong with me? Why can't I go to sleep?" Soon you reach the begging stage. "Please! Oh please, let me sleep." I call this my "Sleepless in Seattle" scenario.

Difficulty going to sleep and staying asleep are two of the most frequent concerns I hear from women in mid-life. Not only do I hear it, I truly empathize with these concerns, because I have experienced them first-hand. Before I went through perimenopause, I never had any trouble falling asleep. When my children were young I was so exhausted I use to dream about sleeping. I could fall asleep standing up! But when I hit perimenopause, my wonderful ability to fall asleep at a moment's notice, left me forever.

You may first notice difficulty falling asleep while transitioning through perimenopause. Difficulty staying asleep

Feelin' Hot?

is one of the hallmark complaints during and after menopause.

No one needs to tell you why a good night's sleep is so important to your health and well-being. You know, that without a restful sleep, your energy level and your moods will suffer. You will be cranky, easily distracted and it may take every ounce of your patience not to snap someone's head off. You don't want to behave this way. This is not you. But after days, weeks and even months of poor quality sleep, your relationships may start to suffer.

Why Can't I Get a Good Night's Sleep?

"I need help sleeping!" "I can't live like this much longer." "What's happening to me?" Women come to me with complaints like this almost daily. Let's talk about what may be contributing to sleep disturbances at mid-life and then we'll discuss solutions.

Three factors contribute to mid-life sleep problems:

1. Age
2. Change in hormone levels
3. Stress

Age. We have no control over our age, so you should expect to experience sleep problems as you approach your mid to late 40s or early 50s.

Change in hormone levels.

Fluctuating hormones levels, particularly estrogen and progesterone during the mid-life transition, can disturb sleep patterns. At the beginning of this book I discussed the decrease in ovulation cycles and how it, in turn, can cause a decrease in three hormones: estrogen, progesterone and testosterone. Well, progesterone plays a key role in helping you fall asleep. During perimenopause the decrease in progesterone may result in an inability for your body to feel drowsy and fall asleep easily.

Estrogen, on the other hand, is the hormone that is responsible for regulating body temperature. Decreasing estrogen levels may cause hot flashes and night sweats. The night sweats may be severe enough to wake you up during the night. When this happens, you may also have difficulty getting back to sleep.

Stress. Stress also contributes to sleep problems. You may feel that you have very little control over the stress in your life, but I am here to tell you that you have more control than you may realize. You have probably lived with enormous stress for so long, you think it is normal. Your body, however, doesn't agree. Your body is your friend and if it could talk, it would tell you that, regardless of societal pressures to multitask, you need to slow down, relax and give your body time to replenish itself. If you listen, your body will tell you when you need to slow down or take a different direction. Shhhh...it's talking to you now. Can you hear it?

Stress: The Adrenal Glands to the Rescue

Your ovaries are one of the organs that release hormones that are important for a good night's sleep. Your adrenal glands are another. The hormones produced by the adrenal glands— adrenaline and cortisol—have been called the "stress" hormones because they are released in response to stress. Prolonged stresses, the kind that you have lived with for several decades, can eventually take its toll on your adrenal glands, reducing their ability to compensate for stress. If your adrenal

Feelin' Hot?

glands are in good working order, however, they will take over for your ovaries after menopause and continue to produce natural estrogen for your body to use.

Healthy adrenal glands create a positive cycle for stress reduction after menopause. A positive cycle looks like this: reduced stress leads to healthy adrenal glands that will provide estrogen after your ovaries quit and, if you have adequate amounts of estrogen available for your body to use, you will probably sleep better, have more energy, be in a good mood, have great relationships and will not have to fret over trying to remember the names of the people you love. So, as you can see, you live in an amazing body.

Sleepless in Seattle—Does it Ever End?

How long will these sleepless nights go on? Women who identify with the "Sleepless in Seattle" scenario described earlier are anxious for an answer to this question. Unfortunately, there is no "cookie-cutter" solution. The precise length of time that is needed for a woman's body to adjust to the changes brought on by aging and menopause varies considerably from individual to individual. Some women breeze through this phase, hardly understanding what the rest of us are talking about. Most women, however, experience changes that last from several months to several years. Now, don't get discouraged. Help is available.

Let's consider some of the practical steps you can take to bring back those "Sweet Dreams." Lifestyle changes and possibly hormone replacement therapy can help restore the quality of sleep you long for. Herbal remedies are also available, if you prefer not to take hormones.

Give Me Hormones!

"Give me some hormones" is a common plea I hear from sleep-deprived women. My girlfriend is on hormones and she says she sleeps like a baby. But will hormones solve your problem? The answer is "Possibly." It is certainly a viable option. When given in the right dosage, hormones have helped provide temporary relief of insomnia, particularly if your hormone levels have been tested and found to be so low they couldn't help put an ant to sleep. Keep in mind, however, that hormones are for temporary relief, meaning that you shouldn't expect to take them for the rest of your life. Judging from the results of the *Women's Health Initiative Study*, hormones are not designed as a life-long habit. Healthy lifestyle choices, however, are a lifetime commitment. As you keep reading, you will learn a lot about making healthy lifestyle choices and the many long-term benefits they provide, without the risks associated with hormones. Magic, hormones are not. A viable temporary option, they are. Another issue to consider is the difference between synthetic and compounding hormones, which I will discuss in detail in Chapter 5, *"Stuck in Hormone Hell."*

The Herbal Option

Herbal therapy is becoming very popular with women as an alternative to hormone replacement therapy. Two herbs, valerian and chamomile have been used to promote sleep. Valerian is a popular, traditional herb that acts like a sedative and is widely used in Europe. Studies on the use of this herb have shown that it may improve the quality of sleep and may even help you fall asleep faster. Chamomile is another herb that has soothing qualities. It can be sipped as a tea, taken in capsule form, or ingested as a liquid extract. Taken right before bed, chamomile may be just the thing to put you in a relaxed mood, all ready for a good night's sleep. Both of these herbs can be found in your nearby health food store or pharmacy.

Neither of these herbs should be taken with alcohol or a sedative. Alcohol may seem like a sedative, but in reality it can have a rebound insomnia effect. In other words, you may fall asleep easily, but you will probably be wake again in a few hours.

Aroma Who?

Another option that is wonderful for relieving tension and relaxing before bed is aromatherapy. I've recently begun experimenting with aromatherapy products myself, and have found them to be a positive, gentle way to prepare my body for restful sleep. What is aromatherapy? Aromatherapy is an ancient therapy that combines the use of aromatic essential oils in order to improve the health and well being of the body, mind and emotions, restoring personal inner balance and harmony. There are several essential oils that are perfect for sleeping difficulties. Lavender, chamomile, orange and neroli work well because of their sedative properties. They can be used in a night-time bath or on your pillow. You may also dab these oils on your temples, the center of your forehead, the back of your neck, and just below your navel, which, according to Ayurvedic practices, are the body's four sleep-related points. Each essential oil has certain emotional and physical benefits. Lavender, for instance, helps relieve nervous tension and stress. It also acts as a healing antiseptic, pain reliever, and anti-inflammatory.

I carry much of my tension in my neck and shoulders. To relieve this tension I recently purchased an aromatherapy comfort wrap. Every night after I have completed my night-time ritual and before I go to bed, I heat up the comfort wrap in the microwave and place it on my pillow. The wrap has been sprayed with lavender. I prop up my book and put on my glasses, and settle in to read quietly for a while. The heat from the wrap feels so soothing to my neck and shoulders and the subtle fragrance from the lavender calms and relaxes every muscle it touches. The good news: I haven't done much reading lately. I feel so good just lying there in my cozy bed. More than once I have found my book in the bed next to me when I wake up in the morning.

Inviting Mr. Sandman to Your Bed Chamber

Many companies manufacture aromatherapy essential oils. I have been using **SwissJust** products imported from Walzenhausen, Switzerland. Although it would probably be a wonderful trip, no, you don't have to go to Switzerland to buy these products. This is the company that I use and one I can highly recommend. The most important point to remember when purchasing aromatherapy essential oils is for the product to be effective for health and well-being, the essential oil must be natural, pure, and of high quality. **SwissJust** has produced and distributed products throughout the world for over 70 years. Their essential oils are 100% natural, and the herbs and extracts are government tested for quality and purity. To find out more about the use of aromatherapy for menopausal symptoms, or for contact information, please refer to the resource section in the back of this book.

This chapter would not be complete without discussing healthy sleeping habits (known in the medical world as sleep hygiene). As your body matures and sleep can no longer be taken for granted, you need to explore new and healthy ways to get a good night's sleep. Assessing your sleep habits and adjusting them, if necessary, should be a part of any therapy you try. The following are a few helpful suggestions:

- Get up and go to bed at about the same time every day, including weekends. Even though I sometimes resist, keeping regular sleep hours has helped me tremendously in improving my sleep habits. When I stick to a sleep schedule, my body takes my desire for a good night's sleep seriously. Another big advantage to training my body for sleep is that now I hardly ever use an alarm clock. I wake up every morning around the same time.
- Avoid caffeine or alcohol within three hours of bedtime.
- Avoid exercise within three hours of bedtime. Exercise can over stimulate your body.
- Try to use the bed only for sleep and sex. Yes, there is sex after menopause! (I use my bed for reading too, even though sleep hygiene specialists consider this a no-no).
- Keep the bedroom quiet, dark, and at a comfortable temperature when you sleep

Now that you know that the bedroom should only be used for sleeping and sex, let's move on and see how you can improve your sex life. *"Where Oh Where Did My Libido Go?"* explores ways to find your libido. And you thought that it was gone forever.

Chapter 4

Where Oh Where Did My Libido Go?

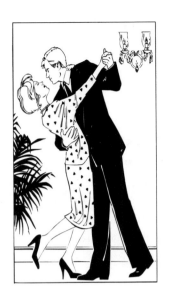

An archaeologist is the best husband a woman can have; the older she gets the more interested he is in her.
— *Agatha Christie*

Has a vital component of your sex life been missing lately? While it could be something as simple as a partner, I'm thinking more along the lines of desire or, using the technical term, libido. In your mother's generation this subject was probably not even covered in a discussion of menopause. But, being baby boomers, we discuss just about everything. Whether we call it sexual desire or libido, many women complain that suddenly it is nowhere to be found. Where did it go? How could it just disappear?

While you maneuver your way through this major transition called menopause, your very wise body is shifting its priorities. It believes that if you are in your middle 40s or early 50s, you couldn't possibly be interested in wanting any more babies. So, to keep you from even thinking about babies, your body shuts down the monthly process of ovulation.

What about women who delayed motherhood until their late 30s or 40s? Some of these women are still able to conceive

Feelin' Hot?

naturally. Others, especially women in their 40s, are able to have children only with the aid of modern medicine. All of these women may still have menopause symptoms with decreased libido while raising children of all ages. Whew! Only a woman could handle all this.

Eventually, all women experience decreasing ovulation cycles resulting in a decreased production of the two "wise women" hormones, estrogen and progesterone, and also the male tag-a-long, testosterone. Testosterone is the hormone that gives you the desire to have sex. While it may seem like your desire to have sex was here yesterday and gone today, in truth your testosterone levels have been slowly decreasing for years.

It doesn't seem quite fair, does it? Here you are in the middle of your life, having accomplished so much in the last two to three decades. You finally feel that you can relax and enjoy life. You and your partner can put the focus on each other. Lately, however, when you look at him, the desire to have sex is just not there. Instead, you may be thinking about cuddling up with a good book!

A Case of Bad Timing

In this new season of your life—one that brings so many physical changes and challenges—the timing seems to be a bit off. Think about it. For the first time in your adult life you are liberated from the worries and bother of pregnancy and menstrual periods, leaving you free to enjoy great sex! Years earlier, when the desire was strong, so were the distractions of using reliable birth control, working around your menstrual cycles and, if you had kids around, securing your bedroom door with a child-proof lock.

So, what do hormones have to do with this dilemma? As it turns out, the hormones that have been in abundance ever since you went through puberty aren't called sex steroids for nothing. You may be thinking that if testosterone is responsible for your desire, and, thanks to menopause, it is now in short supply, just give me testosterone and I will be on my way. If it were that simple, I wouldn't need to devote a whole chapter to libido. There is a lot more to having great sex during and after mid-life than a prescription for testosterone. Like what, you ask? Well, get ready, because we are going to have some fun!

Is He Getting Bigger?

For women a complete scenario must be in place before they have the desire for sex. Most importantly, they must perceive the sexual experience as a positive one that they will look forward to repeating. While testosterone is necessary, it is only a very small part of the overall scenario. In the past, when a woman was going through menopause and mentioned her lack of sexual desire to her doctor, the doctor assumed it was due to vaginal dryness (due to the lack of estrogen) and either prescribed estrogen or suggested the use of a lubricant during intercourse.

It is true that decreasing estrogen levels will leave you less lubricated during sex, because estrogen provides the vaginal lubrication. In fact, the vagina, which is a long muscular tube, requires a bundle of steady estrogen to keep it in good working order. Over time, when your ovaries are no longer providing the same level of estrogen, your vagina starts to shrink in size. This is called "vaginal atrophy." What this really means for you is that without estrogen, the vagina becomes shorter in length, narrower in diameter, and the tissue becomes thin and easily irritated. So what does your male partner make of this shorter, narrower, thinner space? He thinks that all of a sudden he's gotten bigger! So there you have it; once again it's all about him.

So, yes, it is important to provide estrogen to the vagina if lack of lubrication or thinning of the tissue is the problem. But, at best, estrogen only solves part of the difficulty because it fails to address the fundamental problem of desire.

As you can see, good communication between you and your health care provider is a must. Both parties need to be talking about the same issues. Fortunately, the lack-of-desire issue as it pertains to mid-life has been brought into the open on nationally televised talk shows as well as other media. As a result, women and their health care providers are feeling a bit more comfortable discussing it.

As you are now aware, two hormones need to be in place for a woman to have good sex; testosterone, which contributes to desire, and estrogen, which contributes to vaginal lubrication. But as I mentioned earlier, the scenario must be complete for a woman to have good sex. Let's talk about the other components of the scenario.

A Sexual Thought Every 7 to 9 Seconds

Women think about and approach sex differently than men. It's really that basic. It's been said that men have a sexual thought as frequently as every seven to nine seconds (thanks mostly to their high level of testosterone production). I asked my husband if that was true and he said "well maybe not every nine seconds, but many times per day."

Women don't have time to think about sex that often. There are too many other things on our mind that compete for our attention, like the laundry, shopping, paying the bills, what to cook for dinner, arranging social activities for the whole family, our in- laws, why we aren't sleeping, our weight and how we are going to get this all done. Meanwhile a man is probably thinking about two things: work and sex, and not always in that order. As you can see, men and women occupy their minds differently. So even if your doctor gave you a prescription for testosterone or estrogen, you would need to find the time to fill the prescription, and then remember to take the pills. Hopefully, as we put this complex puzzle together, you will see that having good sex—or any sex— after menopause, takes more than just hormones.

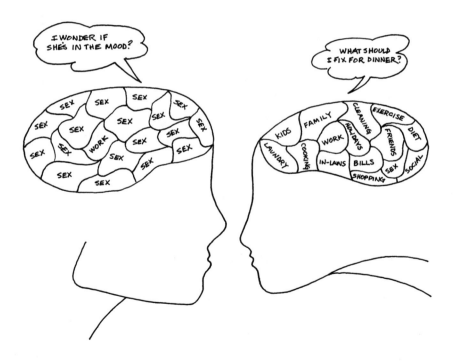

Feelin' Hot?

Time is an essential part of the sex scenario for women. You need time to anticipate sex, to fantasize about sex and, of course, you need time to plan for sex. Most women agree that it's not the physical act of sex that we fantasize about. It's the feeling of intimacy, the romance, and the flirting. And it's the anticipation that our partner will be focused completely on us.

Men, on the other hand, don't need extra time to be in the mood for sex. They have been thinking about it continuously since they went through puberty. While women think about intimacy, men think about the physical sex act. And men are visually motivated. All they need to be stimulated is to see you in front of them-or just a picture of you—and, like clockwork, they are in the mood. What advice do I give men about how to put their "mid-life" women in the mood? If you want to have sex with her in the evening, foreplay needs to start the morning of. And then I go on to redefine foreplay.

Feelings are very important for a woman when it comes to sex. If you have just had an argument with your partner, the last thing you want to do is jump in bed with him. When you decide you are ready to make up with him, it becomes a different story.

So what exactly does it take to increase a woman's desire to have sex after menopause? As I indicated earlier, the puzzle has many pieces.

Testosterone By Itself, Is Not The Answer

Many doctors, in an effort to solve the desire piece of the puzzle, have prescribed estrogen and, more frequently, testosterone. I have tried this approach in my own practice, and have found that it is successful for only a handful of women.

One of the problems with testosterone is that there are very few products to choose from. Being predominantly a male hormone, testosterone products are available in dosages designed for men. These dosages are much too high for women and can cause adverse effects, such as excessive hair growth (in unattractive places), deepening of the voice, and alteration of cholesterol levels, to name a few.

In my professional opinion, the safest testosterone product for women is a compounded testosterone. By compounding a medication [a process that uses natural hormones as opposed to synthetics] there is better control over the strength of the dosage. Also, the dosage can be easily changed if there are adverse effects. This requires a special prescription from your doctor, which must be filled at a compounding pharmacy. I have tried these prescriptions for my patients many times. Sadly, even though this is the safest approach, it has not consistently provided the level or frequency of satisfaction that women desire. When it doesn't work, I am just as disappointed as they are.

To increase my knowledge, I started reading everything I could find on the subject of postmenopausal libido. I also encouraged women to talk about sex and libido in the menopause classes that I was teaching. Actually, they didn't need much encouragement. Over time, and thanks to all the women who have shared their stories, I developed a better picture of what happened to their libido. I don't have all the answers, but I do have some positive solutions that can help women continue to have sex, and better sex, after menopause.

Many factors need to come into focus. As is the case with the whole subject of menopause, one solution is not going to fit every woman. Let's explore the solutions that I have found to see if they will work for you.

Feelin' Hot?

Setting The Stage

Communication is the most important element in any love relationship. I know you've heard this before, but it does bear repeating. If you have experienced a loss of desire to have sex with your partner, you need to tell him. Explain to him, as best you can, that it is not that you don't love him or find him desirable. It's that you just don't think about having sex like you did when you were younger. Don't forget to explain that the loss of hormones contributes significantly to the situation. Men take your "loss of desire" very personally. They equate frequency of sex with love. When the frequency of sex diminishes, they think love has diminished as well. If you don't feel comfortable talking about this with your partner, ask him to read this chapter first and then the two of you can discuss it.

Just think...once you have discussed your lack of desire with your partner and explained its cause, the situation is out in the open. No more pretending or avoiding situations that may lead to sex when you aren't ready for it. You have now set the stage for a positive approach to finding a solution that will involve both of you.

Is It Your Intention to Once Again Have Great Sex?

Before even attempting to deal with lack of libido, you must become clear about your intentions. Intention is a powerful word that refers to what one hopes to achieve or attain. A clear intention to attain a goal generates energy with a laser-like focus. If you intend to once again have great sex, you will. In other words, make up your mind that having sex is important to you and that you are willing to put the necessary thought and energy into getting it.

Clarity regarding our intentions is a wonderful gift. Once we are clear, we then move naturally and almost effortlessly in the right direction. So if your intention is to continue to have great sex with your partner, step one is to communicate your intention to him.

At this point you are probably thinking, "Great. My intention is to have great sex with my partner, and I have communicated this to him, explaining all the reasons why I haven't been thinking about sex lately. Now, how am I supposed to get in the mood?" First, you are going to plan for it, and then you will practice the plan. You need to include your partner in the planning too, so you're both on the same page. You will then repeat the plan, perfecting it as you go. Don't worry; I'm going to show you how.

A Date With Your Libido

First and foremost, you need to start from wherever you are. By this I mean that if you and your partner haven't had sex for a while, say weeks, months or years, you won't go from no sex to great sex overnight. You need to take a few basic steps first. If you are still having sex, but not as frequently as you once did, you can move along a little faster.

I am going to first assume that you enjoy sex with your partner and that your body functions well sexually, meaning that you are well lubricated and achieve orgasm. Orgasm may take a little longer to achieve than it once did, but don't get discouraged. With patience and the right technique, it can still happen. The problem is that you just don't think about sex anymore so, unless your partner initiates it, it just doesn't happen.

Your plan will be "Create the Perfect Sex Date." Here's how you do it. Pick a day of the week when you and your partner can spend the evening together. Write in your daily planner or calendar under that day: Sex date with Jack (insert correct name). Start planning the date one week in advance. Don't forget to have Jack put it on his calendar as well. Have an agreement that unless there is a real emergency, neither of you may cancel. Every day for one week leading up to your date with Jack, write on your calendar or to-do list: Saturday Night, The Perfect Sex Date. This will stimulate your brain to start anticipating the arrival of the day, the evening and the final moment. If you practice thinking about the upcoming evening every day for the week leading up to the date, the anticipation alone will stimulate thoughts of how good it used to feel to make love to your partner. Sometimes all you need is a little reminding.

Next, you get to plan the evening. It can involve anything that you and your partner enjoy doing together, like dinner at your favorite restaurant, or perhaps a night of dancing or listening to your favorite jazz band while enjoying cocktails and watching the sunset. If you love to cook, (after all these years) picture yourself making his favorite dinner and cuddling on the sofa watching a video. Let your mind wander. This is your date to create.

Every day for the entire week leading up to the date you will have delicious thoughts about the big night, just the two of you, together. Every time you see him or hear his voice, look at him a little differently with the thought in mind of spending a whole evening together, away from the distractions of everyday life. Even though you may have been together forever, try to remember how you felt when you first started seeing each other. Recall the anticipation and excitement you once felt when planning for a date together. Don't get discouraged if the feeling seems to be gone, never to return, because I am here to tell you that it is just in hiding. With a little coaxing on your part, this feeling will quickly come out of its hiding place. You have it; you just forgot where you put it.

On the morning of the date start anticipating the evening. Picture candlelight and music, and how it will feel to have his full attention. Think about it every chance you get during the day. Don't plan too many activities the day of your date. You don't want to be exhausted. If the date is outside the house and you need time to get ready, schedule that time into your day. Start by taking a warm, relaxing bath. If you are feeling a little stressed, add aromatherapy essential oils to the bath water. A little lavender or melissa will help you relax and enjoy the moment. Follow the bath with your favorite moisturizing lotion. Pamper yourself. This is your time to attend to every wonderful detail. When you dress for the evening, wear the outfit in your closet that always brings you compliments. You have one, I'm sure of it!

A woman knows she's wearing the right dress,
when her man wants to take it off!
— Robert Paul

And Finally, The Date Has Arrived

During the date, keep the focus on each other. Don't take your partner to a place where he will be easily distracted. For my husband, I would not pick a place with views of boats, trains or airplanes. These items quickly put him in a trance. During the evening focus on conversation that is fun and light. This is not the time to bring up controversial issues that may lead to heated discussions. Remember, you are going

Feelin' Hot?

to make love to this man when the time comes.

Finally, the time has come. The moment that you have anticipated for a week has arrived. Remember, your partner probably didn't need the whole week to think about it. He was ready when you told him to put it on his calendar.

Congratulations! If your intention was clear, you communicated your intentions to your partner and you followed through with the plan, I can only imagine what a wonderful night it was. If it was perfect in every way, just repeat the process and the plan, changing the details to prevent boredom. Your desire will never be in question again.

You may be thinking that this sounds like a lot of work. But remember, anytime you try something new and unfamiliar the process feels awkward at first. With every successful date that you and your partner have, you will both want to repeat the process. Over time it will become easier and easier to plan. Take turns creating the date. Let your partner plan a perfect date for the two of you. You will be pleasantly surprised at what he comes up with. No pun intended.

In a perfect world, when a woman complains of a lack of desire while transitioning through menopause, the solution may simply be learning how to put sex back into a healthy, loving, relationship. I mentioned earlier that in order for the above solutions to work, the body must respond appropriately as well. For some women having great sex after menopause is not as simple as putting it on your calendar. Physical problems like insufficient vaginal lubrication or a delayed or absent orgasmic response may be the culprit. When this is the case, many women feel that it's not worth the effort, and that eating chocolate brings just as much pleasure. However, as pleasurable as eating chocolate might be, it is a solo experience, one that will not improve intimacy with your partner.

Sometimes couples need a review and a little coaching on different techniques to find that orgasm. Delayed or absent orgasmic response may have a physiological basis or possibly a psychological basis, the discussion of which becomes more complicated, and requires a more thorough investigation by a trained professional. Whatever the situation may be for you, if you truly want more intimacy and better sex with your partner, I support your efforts and encourage you not to give up. Remember, menopause is a major change in our life, but it is not the end.

Let's move on to the chapter everyone has been waiting for. We'll discuss the role that hormones, or lack of them, play in this complex puzzle called menopause.

Chapter 5

Stuck in Hormone Hell

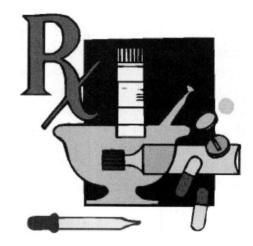

Hormones!
Hormones!
Hormones!

You can't live with them and you can't live without them...or can you?

Who's Driving This Hormone Bus?

These days you can't go near a women's magazine, a newspaper or the evening news without encountering yet another alarming discussion or editorial regarding hormone replacement therapy. If you are anything like my patients, friends, colleagues and family members, you have probably reached a highly informed state of...confusion.

Should you start taking hormones or stop taking them? If you start them, how long should you stay on them? Should you take synthetic or compounded hormones? How does your doctor or health care practitioner decide which one to prescribe? And what's the difference, anyway? And when you finally decide what to take, how do you decide what form to take it in—a pill, a patch, a cream, a ring, or a lozenge? Is there a test you can take to figure it all out? And if there is, why hasn't someone offered it to you!

Who's driving this hormone bus anyway?

Let's start with a crash course in hormones. By definition, a hormone is a substance produced by one organ, which is then sent via the blood stream to a target organ where it stimulates that organ to perform its function. Sound complicated? To put it another way, a hormone is a chemical messenger that targets a designated organ and stimulates it to function according to its design. Without hormones to spur activity, our organs would probably lie around all day and do nothing.

Your ovaries require specific hormones to stimulate them to produce other hormones that make you the awesome woman that you are. There you have it. It's that simple. Well, actually, the role of hormones in your body is a rather complex subject. But, I'm sure you get the picture.

When you went through puberty your hormones were functioning in their finest fashion, acting as agents of extraordinary change in your body. You transformed from a little girl into a lovely young woman. You developed breasts, and probably begged your mother for a training bra. You developed hips and could finally keep a straight skirt up. There were also those pimples, pubic hair and, off in the distant future, a prom dress to think about.

Pregnancy is another time in a woman's life when hormones, in the right amounts, bring about the extraordinary...a new little person. For the past four decades or so a unique package of hormones when in the right amount and in perfect balance has delivered your regular monthly

Feelin' Hot?

periods. If you ever experienced PMS symptoms however this was a sign that your hormones were somewhat out of balance. And now, menopause brings another time in a woman's life when hormones become out of balance. As you can see, hormones are very important to a woman's body.

Why All the Confusion Then?

The confusion began when medical science started exploring ways to help women continue the benefits of hormones after their bodies stopped producing them. After all, why give up on a good thing?

Then pharmaceutical companies got wind of the medical research and saw the commercial viability of mass-producing and marketing hormones to aging women. And before you could say "testosterone," the market was so flooded with different brands and types of hormones that the days of going solo through menopause were a horror story from the distant past (pre-1950s).

Pharmaceutical companies, through aggressive and well-funded marketing strategies, have convinced doctors, health care professionals and, most importantly, women that hormone replacement is necessary if women expect to live long and healthy lives. Advertising campaigns have successfully persuaded women that hormones are the magic elixir that will keep them looking and feeling young as long as they continue taking them. And even if you are not concerned with looking younger, you could still be taken in by claims that hormones will protect you from heart disease and keep you from being hunched over in a wheel chair due to weakened bones.

You Are Not Alone

You are not the only one who bought into this message. We, the medical profession, bought into it first! Then we passed the message on to you. We thought we were doing a good thing. Despite conflicting evidence from scientific trials as to the overall benefit for most women, we still believed that the benefits far outweighed the risks.

Hormones have been available and widely prescribed to women since the 1950s. Through trial and error we've learned a great deal about the benefits and the risks that come with hormone replacement therapy. So, who has been driving the hormone replacement bus? Well, it has been driven by a combination of pharmaceutical companies, the medical community and, last but never least, the consumer.

So what are the benefits and risks of taking hormones and how do you decide if you need them? Read on...

Hormones provide many benefits to women going through menopause. We have already discussed the uncomfortable physical and emotional symptoms you may experience during this transition such as hot flashes, vaginal dryness, mood swings, sleep disturbances, irregular periods, memory changes, and decreased libido. Taking hormones will relieve many of these symptoms, particularly hot flashes and vaginal dryness. Research has also shown that hormones, especially estrogen, help reduce bone loss, which some women experience after menopause. On the other hand, there are risks associated with hormone replacement therapy including increased rates of breast cancer, blood clots, heart attacks, strokes, endometrial cancer and gall bladder disease. And recently, dementia was added to the list.

So, how do you decide if you should take hormones? And how does your doctor decide whether you need them? Until the Women's Health Initiative study came out in 2002, most doctors and health care professionals suggested that any woman who did not have a medical reason not to take hormones, (i.e. a history of breast cancer or blood clots or gall bladder disease) should consider taking them for their supposedly long-term benefits such as protection from osteoporosis and heart disease. The Women's Health Initiative, the largest randomized clinical trial involving 16,608 postmenopausal women, found that women who used a combination of Conjugated Equine Estrogen (Premarin) and Medroxyprogesterone acetate (Provera) daily had a greater incidence of invasive breast cancer, heart attacks, blood clots and strokes. On the positive side, there were fewer occurrences of hip fractures and less diagnosed colon cancer among those women during the five years of this trial.

Due to the results of the Women's Health Initiative study, the whole prescribing picture has changed. And, in my opinion, it has changed for the better. Why? Because now, women know hormones are not the magic elixir. Hormones alone cannot give you the health and longevity you desire. You still need to practice healthy lifestyle choices, especially a balanced diet and daily exercise. Then you can consider the possibility of adding short-term hormone replacement therapy to get you through the rough spots during the menopause transition.

I know, I know: please, not the exercise word. Yes, the exercise word. You are reading this book because you want to know the truth about menopause. If I told you that you could sail through the rest of your life in the best of health without exercising, I would not be telling you the truth. I will talk about the importance of exercise in the chapters that follow. Right now let's get back to hormones.

Should I Take Hormones?

So, how do you decide if you should take hormones? Symptoms are the first thing to consider. Ask yourself the following:

- Am I having symptoms that impact the quality of my day-to-day life?
- Am I having hot flashes that I can't live with another minute?
- Am I having vaginal dryness that is painful with or without sex?
- Am I having mood swings that affect me and the people around me?
- Am I having sleepless nights?

If you answered yes to the majority of these questions, you may want to consider short-term hormone replacement therapy. Symptoms—not the prevention of health conditions that you don't yet have—are the reason to consider hormone replacement; symptoms that you can't tolerate another minute. And then, only if you've thoroughly discussed your situation with your health care provider or doctor.

If, after an honest self-assessment, you decide to try hormones, the question becomes which kind should you try. As you may know, you have several choices.

Natural and Synthetic Hormones

Synthetic Hormones. The most commonly prescribed hormones are those produced synthetically by pharmaceutical companies. The reason these hormones are called synthetic is because:

1) they are commercially produced in large quantities in predetermined doses, and

2) they are manmade, which means, the molecular structure of the estrogen and progesterone used in combination or separately have been altered from the naturally occurring estrogen and progesterone produced by the ovaries. This allows the pharmaceutical company to obtain a patent from the Food and Drug Administration (FDA).

You have probably heard of an estrogen called Premarin and a progestin (synthetic progesterone) called Provera. These two products in combination have been the most frequently prescribed hormone therapy in the United States. The Women's Health Initiative used this combination, which is called PremPro, in their recent clinical study. Since the development of this combination, many other pharmaceutical companies have come up with their own version of estrogen and progestin combinations, including Activella and Femhrt. The difference between PremPro and these other products is the kinds of estrogen and progestin used. All three products are synthetic, manmade substances. There are many other estrogens and progestins on the market that can be used in combination to accomplish the same result. And this is only the tip of the iceberg. Whew! Can you see where this can get complicated?

So, how does your doctor decide which combination to give you? And why do you need to take estrogen and progesterone (or its synthetic version, progestin) in combination? This is where marketing and costs come in to play. If you are not restricted by your insurance company dictating how much you can spend for a prescriptive drug, the doctor will usually prescribe what he or she feels most comfortable with, meaning that hormone combination which the majority of patients have experienced the greatest results (symptom relief) with the fewest side effects.

If your uterus is intact (you have not had a hysterectomy), you will always need progesterone, or its manmade version, progestin, to offset the effects of estrogen on the endometrial lining of the uterus. One of the responsibilities of estrogen is to build up the lining of the uterus in preparation for a pregnancy. Each month that you don't become pregnant, progesterone causes the lining of the uterus to withdraw and, whala, your period arrives. If you don't have enough progesterone—or in the case of hormone replacement therapy, a progestin—to offset the buildup of the lining in the uterus caused by estrogen, the estrogen can lead to trouble in the uterus, i.e., possible cancer, known in the medical community as endometrial carcinoma. Who would have ever thought a woman's body could be so complicated?

Compounded (or Natural) Hormones.

Fortunately, synthetic hormones are not your only choice. Compounded hormones are another way to go. Compounded—or bio-identical hormones—are becoming much more popular in the eyes of consumers because they have fewer side effects than the synthetics. Why? The estrogen and progesterone in the compounded formula is in its natural, unchanged form. The chemist takes wild yam and soy and, through a chemical process, creates the three types of estrogens along with the one and only type of progesterone that your ovaries produce. Yes, that's right. Your ovaries produce estrogen in three different forms: estradiol, estrone and estriol.

A compounding pharmacist can make up all three forms for you. When your doctor writes a prescription for compounded hormones, he or she must specify if one, two or all three forms of estrogen will be present in the prescription. With compounding hormones you have a choice as to what type of estrogen is in the prescription. With synthetically produced hormones, the pharmaceutical company predetermines everything.

Where Do I Get a Compounded Prescription Filled?

Not every pharmacy or pharmacist can fill a prescription for compounded hormones. You must find a pharmacy that has the expertise to perform the specialized procedure necessary to fill a compounded prescription. The benefit of going to the additional trouble is that the prescription can be individualized to the needs of each woman. Compounded hormones are not mass-produced and are *not patentable*, which explains why large pharmaceutical companies are not in the compounding business. Each individual prescription is unique to each individual woman. It is similar to a popular fast food restaurant slogan; "We don't make it until you order it!"

The down side of compounded hormones is that many insurance companies do not cover the cost of these prescriptions. Are you beginning to see why the subject of hormone therapy is so complicated?

Compounded or Synthetic: Which Form Is Right For Me?

So how do you choose between synthetic hormones and compounded hormones? By now, you know better than to expect a simple answer. Here's the bottom line: The traditional medical community is not as familiar with compounded hormones as they are with synthetic. This is due to two factors.

1) Pharmaceutical companies devote a lot of money to marketing synthetic hormones, which makes doctors feel comfortable prescribing them.

2) Due to the lack of large clinical trials of compounded hormones, the traditional medical community does not feel comfortable prescribing them. The studies that have been done so far on compounded hormones are smaller (not as many women in them) and are not generally published in the kind of medical journals the majority of doctors read. As a result, what little education doctors have about compounded hormones comes largely from the consumer. And while word-of-mouth advertising is powerful, it is a very slow process.

The best way for you to decide between synthetic and compounded hormones is to examine your beliefs and preferences, and listen to your intuition. Educate yourself as much as possible about the differences between the two by reading, attending classes that may be offered at your local hospital, talking to compounding pharmacists, and, of course, consulting with your doctor. Pharmacists who fill compounded prescriptions are an excellent resource. The resource section of this book includes information on how to contact a compounded pharmacist in your area.

I have a trusted pharmacist that I consult with who specializes in compounded hormones for women going through menopause. I consult with her frequently when I prescribe compounded hormones for my patients. She has opened my eyes and expanded my knowledge of both synthetically made hormones and those that are compounded. I have also had the benefit of observing how women respond to synthetically made hormones versus compounded hormones. I still believe, however, that a hormone is a hormone is a hormone, regardless of its form.

The decision you make about hormones should be a considered, educated one. Let your health history, your beliefs about hormones and your symptoms guide you toward a wise decision. Either form of hormones will probably relieve your symptoms. What you want is whatever form of hormone that will give you the greatest relief with the least side effects or, ideally, no side effects at all.

I am often asked which of the two hormone forms is safer. The answer, unfortunately, is that no one really knows for sure. This is what makes the discussion of hormones so frustrating. It seems logical to assume that a hormone in its natural, unchanged molecular state—in this case a compounded hormone—is safer. But until we have more information, we must assume that all hormones, synthetic or compounded, carry the same risks.

Do I Have to Take a Pill?

Most doctors prescribe hormones in the form of a pill. Hormones, however, are also available in patches, creams, rings, vaginal tablets, and lozenges. Which vehicle you want to use largely depends on your preference. Consider convenience, because you won't get consistent relief from your symptoms unless you are consistent in taking the hormones. Before the Women's Health Initiative released its study results the recommended dosage was the same for every woman. Many women found this universal approach surprising. When you stop and think about it, if we are all unique and different, how can one dosage be right for all of us?

Determining Dosage

You may wonder why your doctor doesn't test your hormone levels routinely before prescribing hormones. While it seems logical, the level range that is considered normal is so wide that it is difficult to correctly interpret hormone levels from blood samples. Doctors and health practitioners rely heavily on your description of symptoms to determine when, what kind, and how much of a hormone to give you.

Here's a little more information about how hormones work. The sex hormones in your body are carried throughout your blood stream via carrier proteins, which can be compared to a hitch-hiker hitching a ride on the back of a motorcycle. However, certain hormones called "free hormones" do not attach to carrier proteins. These free hormones are available to relieve your menopausal symptoms.

Blood sampling cannot distinguish between free hormones and the ones delivered via carrier proteins. It measures only total hormone levels and can't be used to determine how much free hormone is available for use in your tissue.

Saliva testing, however, can measure the amount of free hormones in your body. Your salivary glands only allow the free hormones to enter into the saliva. By collecting and analyzing saliva samples the levels of your free hormones can be determined.

While this type of testing has been around for some time, it is not available at the labs used by most medical doctors, and is, therefore, still new to them. The cost of this testing may or may not be covered by your insurance. Information about saliva testing can be found at your local compounding pharmacy. I have also included information about it in the resource section in the back of this book.

Two final questions remain regarding hormone use.

- How long should you stay on hormones?
- If you are already on hormones, should you stop?

The recommendation on how long a woman should stay on hormones was revised after the results of the Women's Health Initiative study were released in July 2002. The revised recommendation advises women to limit hormone use to three to five years. It also advises women to take the lowest dose necessary to relieve symptoms. Remember, this is only a recommendation. You will still need to consult with your doctor. How long you decide to stay on hormones must be determined by your individual needs and medical situation.

If you've been on hormones for more than five years, you are undoubtedly wondering if you should stop taking them. In July 2002, help lines in gynecology offices around the world started ringing off the hook and haven't stopped since. As you might have guessed by now, easy answers are not to be had. You must measure the benefits that you receive from hormone replacement therapy against the long-term risk associated with its use. Many women have clearly stated that hormones make them feel so much better that they are willing to take whatever risks come with their continued use.

As I have stated many times, every woman is unique. It is important to have your doctor inform you of your individual risks. Then you can make the decision that is best for you. If you decide to stop taking hormones, I would advise you to taper off slowly rather than going cold turkey. Your body needs a winding down period. Women who stop cold turkey often experience a sudden, unpleasant resurgence of symptoms. When you have been free from daily hot flashes for years, you are not happy when they show up again! Your body reacts similarly when the sugar or caffeine to which it has become accustomed is suddenly cut off. A slow tapering off can be accomplished by either reducing the hormone dosage each day, or by reducing the number of days each week that you take them. This gradual method allows your body to adjust slowly to the reduced amount of hormones available to keep you in balance.

By now, you may find you are curious about alternatives to hormone replacement therapy. Follow me now as I introduce you to new ways of managing your menopause symptoms. The next chapter, *"Every Woman Loves a Compliment"* (even though compliment is spelled differently), will open your realm of choices even wider.

Feelin' Hot?

Chapter 6

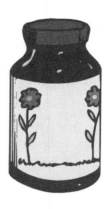

Every Woman Loves a Compliment

Don't tell a woman she's pretty; tell her there's no other woman like her, and all roads will open to you.
— Jules Renard

When was the last time you were paid a genuine compliment? You know, the kind that is given sincerely from the heart, the kind that leaves you glowing all day long.

While compliments of this nature always make us feel better they do not take away our menopause symptoms. A *complement* however, might. Complement spelled with an "e" rather than an "i" refers to the act of completing, as when the color of your dress complements your eyes or when your new exercise program complements your commitment to a healthier lifestyle. Synonymous terms include: interrelated, interconnected, interdependent, companion.

Hormone Alternatives

As the safety of hormone replacement therapy continues to be questioned, many women are looking for substances other than hormones (alternatives), or substances with hormones (complements) that will provide benefits without introducing additional risks.

If you decide to explore this area, your preferences and personal beliefs will help guide you through your choices. It is important to acknowledge and honor them as part of the decision-making process.

Let's begin with an understanding of the differences between complementary/alternative medicine and conventional medicine. Simply stated, conventional medicine or therapies are those that are widely practiced and accepted by the mainstream medical community. Also referred to as Western, modern and mainstream, conventional medicine is practiced by most medical doctors (MDs), ODs (doctors of osteopathy) and health care practitioners. Most of these medical specialists attend the same conferences, prescribe the same medicine and read the same medical journals.

Complementary and alternative medicine, also referred to as integrative medicine, includes a wide variety of healing philosophies, approaches, and therapies that conventional medicine does not commonly use, accept, understand, study or make available. A therapy is usually called complementary when it is used in addition to or in conjunction with conventional treatment. It is called alternative when it is used instead of conventional treatment.

Complementary and Alternative Approaches

Complementary and alternative medicine may include a variety of "natural health products" such as herbal products, vitamin and mineral supplements, and homeopathic medicines, as well as traditional Chinese medicine. A report released in 2000 by the National Institute of Health (NIH) found that approximately one-third of Americans and more than 50 percent of Canadians use "natural health products." It is now 2003 and I would bet that if the NIH did another study, the number would be even higher.

As consumer interest in alternatives grows, the shelves in the stores that sell them are overflowing. The claims they make for relief of every imaginable symptom can make your head spin. How do you decide which product to take? You may also wonder why your doctor or healthcare practitioner hasn't advised you in this area, or recommended a particular over-the-counter product.

Conventional medical doctors have a very limited knowledge of the use and benefits of over-the-counter herbs, vitamins and dietary supplements. Since medical schools don't include alternative medicine in their curriculum, doctors are not educated to the benefits of so-called "natural" products. And, because the FDA does not regulate any product that you can buy over the counter, medical doctors are concerned about the safety and purity of these products.

Belief systems come into play for physicians as well. Conventional medical doctors are heavily invested in standard medical-school traditions. These traditions maintain that conventional medicine is the only proven way to heal the body. The proof, which is derived from scientific trials, is called evidence-based medicine. Evidence-based medicine is the gold standard by which conventional medicine is practiced.

But as consumers begin to question this belief and confront their physicians, many health care practitioners are now open to learning more about over-the-counter products, as well as how other cultures deal with the menopausal transition.

What About Herbs?

There are many alternative choices to relieve menopausal symptoms and they are readily available at your local health food store, or nearby food market. Let's take a common menopause symptom: hot flashes.

Black cohosh is an herb that many women have tried, with some success, to improve moods and relieve hot flashes. The most popular black cohosh presently being sold in a standardized form is called Remifemin. Standardized means that the herb is in a pure-grade form; no other additives are mixed with the black cohosh. When choosing an over-the-counter herb, find one that is standardized, which assures you of getting the highest grade available, which in turn will give you the best chance of experiencing symptom relief. Also, keep in mind that over-the-counter herbs generally take longer to produce results than conventional, prescribed medication. The reason for this is unclear. Patience is an important virtue when trying any new product. It is unlikely that any herbal product is going to work over night.

Other herbs that are gaining in popularity include red clover, St. John's wort, gingko biloba, valerian, kava, ginseng, and dong quai. Most of these herbs have been around for centuries and have been used successfully in other cultures. Which herb you use depends on your symptom. Here is a summary of the most common herbs.

Red clover was originally used by Native Americans to treat whooping cough, gout and cancer. Recently, red clover extracts have been promoted to relieve the menopausal symptoms of hot flashes and vaginal dryness. Proponents claim that its effectiveness comes from its estrogenic effects. But research results have been disappointing.

St. John's wort has been used to treat mild to moderate depression.

Gingo biloba is popular as a memory enhancer. Almost every menopausal woman could use a boost in her memory. The interaction that is supposed to occur from using Gingo biloba is to dilate blood vessels thereby increasing circulation to the brain. Some researchers believe with increased circulation to the brain there will be an improvement in memory.

Valerian may help some women who are bothered by menopause-related sleep problems.

Kava has been used to relieve anxiety, although recently it has been linked to liver failure and cirrhosis in reports from Germany, Switzerland and the United States. It has been banned in several European countries and Canada, but it is still available in the United States.

Ginseng has long had a prominent place in traditional Chinese medicine. Despite its popularity with the Chinese, ginseng has not been found effective in treating hot flashes or any other symptoms associated with menopause.

Dong quai is another common component of traditional Chinese medicine. Studies done on dong quai have not proven its effectiveness in relieving hot flashes or other menopausal symptoms either. Critics of these studies point out that Chinese herbs are not usually administered alone, and therefore beneficial effects may only result from combination of herbs used by Chinese practitioners.

So, once again the question becomes…

What's A Woman to Do?

After describing these herbs it would seem natural for me to provide advice on dosage—how much, how often and for how long. But, because I am not an expert in the use of alternative therapies, I'm going to leave that to a professional practitioner.

Personally, I do believe that alternatives are a viable option for women. I find the study of these less conventional approaches fascinating and I learn more each day. I also believe that to derive the greatest benefit from them with the least chance of side effects, a woman wishing to try natural alternatives should be referred to a competent practitioner who specializes in prescribing these products.

The last thing you want to do is go to your nearby health food store and ask the 17-year-old male clerk which product he recommends for hot flashes or memory loss. First, I'm sure he has no idea and, second, should you develop side effects like abnormal bleeding, he is not going to be able to help you. Additionally, you can spend lots of money trying to find the right product with the right blend that takes care of your symptoms.

A naturopath or herbalist, on the other hand, has studied herbs and other substances found in nature. By taking a careful history of your symptoms he or she will know which herb will most likely work for you, saving you countless hours of research as well as some hard-earned money. And you will have your expert's support as well as his or her expert advice.

The Word On Vitamins and Dietary Supplementation

What About Soy?

In addition to herbs and vitamin supplementation, the introduction of products with soy into the diet is quickly gaining popularity with women in mid-life. Soy is a plant-based protein and is a weak natural source of estrogen. There is some evidence that eating soy foods such as tofu may be helpful in reducing hot flashes. Studies of different cultures reveal that Japanese women have very few complaints about hot flashes. Many researchers attribute this to the prevalence of soy in the Japanese diet. It's a staple food for Japanese women. Since soy is plant-based, it is a better source of protein than animal protein, and studies are showing that soy may lower your risk of heart disease. Whenever possible it is always better to get the nutrients that soy provides from the food you eat, rather than from a supplement because the body absorbs the nutrients more efficiently.

Vitamin Supplements – Another Option

Vitamins and minerals are important at any age. But, as you get older they may play an important role in disease prevention. Did you know that your body needs more than 45 vitamins and minerals to maintain your health? There is a small amount of evidence that vitamin E provides at least some relief from hot flashes. Some vitamin and mineral supplements can help reduce the risk of various age-related chronic illnesses. Let's take calcium as an example.

Calcium maintains proper functioning in the bones, heart, and nerves. Many women may begin to lose bone mass at a rapid pace around menopause. That makes it even more important during and after menopause to get an adequate amount of calcium. But calcium can't do it alone; calcium and vitamin D work together to maintain bone density. It is recommended that if you are not taking hormone replacement therapy, you should get at least 1500mg of calcium with vitamin D in your diet each day. The best source of dietary calcium is in dairy products. But calcium is also found in dark leafy green vegetables, dried beans, nuts and fortified foods. Studies have also shown that most women only get around 600mg of calcium from the food that they eat. So calcium should be on your list of important supplements to take each day. It is best to take calcium supplements in divided doses of no more than 500mg. This assures that the calcium you take is well absorbed and not wasted.

The **B vitamins** should also be on your list. Maintaining appropriate levels of certain B vitamins can help ward off anemia, depression, insomnia, irritability, and possibly heart disease. B vitamins should be taken together as a B complex in order to achieve the best balance. Folic acid, or folate, is a B vitamin with a variety of healthful properties. You may have heard that women who are pregnant need to take folic acid to help prevent neural tube defects in their developing fetuses. As it turns out, folic acid may help lower your risks for several types of cancer, including breast cancer and colon cancer. In particular, a daily supplement with folic acid helps reduce cancer risks in people who drink alcohol. Folate is found in green leafy vegetables and oranges. Folic acid is the form of folate that's found in supplements and fortified cereals. The recommended daily dose is 400mcg (micrograms) per day. Make sure your multivitamin contains at least 3 milligrams of vitamin B6, 6 milligrams of vitamin B12, and 400 micrograms of folate.

Dietary intake of vitamin B12, B6 and folate may also help to combat an elevated level of homocysteine. Homocysteine is an amino acid that is found in the blood of people who eat high amounts of animal protein. High levels of homocysteine can cause inflammation in arteries, which in turn puts you at a higher risk for heart disease. Heart disease is the number one cause of death among women over the age of 50.

Feelin' Hot?

Where Did Those Free Radicals Go?

The discussion of vitamin supplementation as you age would not be complete without mentioning antioxidants, which capture and neutralize free radicals that damage cells in the body. Three vitamins are considered to have the highest antioxidant properties:

- Vitamin E
- Vitamin C
- Beta-carotene

Vitamin E has been shown to relieve hot flashes in breast cancer survivors. Even though randomized, controlled studies don't support taking antioxidant supplements as a way of preventing chronic diseases, population studies do. People who eat more whole grains, fruits and vegetables that are high in antioxidants have shown to have lower rates of heart disease than those who eat less of these foods.

Vitamin C is another important vitamin that keeps our skin, eyes, and gums healthy; it also helps ward off infection. Some encouraging evidence shows that women with diets that contain more vitamin C have stronger bones. Many luscious foods contain plenty of vitamin C, including bananas, cantaloupe, strawberries and, of course, citrus fruits. Examples of vitamin C-rich vegetables include broccoli, peppers, asparagus, cauliflower and tomatoes. Even potatoes contain significant amounts of vitamin C. The point is that you can easily get an adequate amount of vitamins from the foods you eat, without having to rely on supplements.

Beta carotene, which is another important antioxidant, also helps ward off heart disease and other chronic illnesses, and can be found in abundance in all the fruits and vegetables mentioned above, as well as carrots.

Let's Not Forget Aromatherapy

Aromatherapy, as I mentioned earlier, is fast becoming a favorite of mine for the relief of menopausal symptoms. The more I learn about the essential oils involved in aromatherapy, the more I realize how valuable they are as a "complement" to help maintain health and vigor throughout all periods of life. The subtle yet powerful oils can reduce menopausal symptoms from hot flashes, mood swings, sleep disturbances, fuzzy thinking and decreased energy, lulling you into calmness and relaxation. Use essential oils of pure grade for the most effective results. Complementary and alternative therapies also include a variety of body treatments. A soothing massage, acupressure and acupuncture, as well as tai chi, yoga and daily stretching, will bring countless benefits to your body during this transitional time in your life.

As you can see, no single alternative product or therapy will benefit every woman. If you get only one thing out of this book, let it be this: No single size, treatment, dosage or method will fit all. You may need to try several different products and a combination of different approaches before you find the one that works for you. Try not to get discouraged or expect overnight success with any one product. A strong and consistent commitment to your health is your best bet for success.

Many women complain that their weight goes up, up, up during the transition to menopause. Let's find out what's going on and how you can have better control over your weight as you age.

Feelin' Hot?

Chapter 7

Weight No More

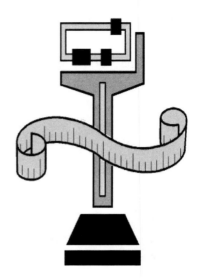

Thank you for calling the Weight Loss Hotline. If you'd like to lose a half pound right now, press 1 eighteen thousand times.
— Randy Glasbergen

Life sure is funny sometimes. For years the popular press bombarded you with how-to articles; how to have a slimmer body, how to have a sexy body; how to look 20 years younger. Most of these articles told you to focus on your weight. So you consulted the weight charts to find your proper height/weight ratio; if you are yea tall, you should weigh yea much.

New Diet Step 1: Weigh yourself (oh God)
New Diet Step 2: Find your ideal weight on the chart
New Diet Step 3: Embark upon a tortuous period of deprivation to reconcile your weight to your height.

You were kept going by the thought of that day when the scale finally registered your perfect weight. That blissful day when you would look as smashing in your wardrobe as you expected to the day you put down your credit card. That day of soaring self-confidence, when your lucky partner would finally have the sex kitten of his dreams.

But…now that you are maneuvering through menopause you acknowledge that the sex kitten dream is a bit dated. Still, you would like your acquired maturity and wisdom to be complemented by a sleek, desirable body, and oh, how you would love to look smashing in your clothes.

Calculating a Healthy Weight

Several things have changed in the billion-dollar-a-year weight loss industry. The experts have shifted their emphasis from the simple height/weight chart to the more complex body-mass index chart and waist/hip ratio measurements. What does your waist/hip ratio measurement have to do with anything?

This calculation is supposed to predict how long you are going to live without major diseases like heart disease and diabetes. Studies have shown that men or women who carry the majority of their fat around their waist and abdominal area are more frequently diagnosed with diabetes and heart disease. As you will remember, heart disease is the number one killer of women over the age of 50. Women who have diabetes are at a higher risk of heart disease. When you carry the majority of your fat around your waist and abdomen you are said to have an apple shape. If the majority of your fat is around your hips you are a pear shape. A pear shape does not carry the same medical significance. So how do you determine your waist/hip ratio? First measure your hips in inches, and

Feelin' Hot?

then measure your waist in inches. Then divide the hip measurement into the waist measurement. (Where did I put that calculator?) Does any of this make sense?

If you are like most of the 40 million women in the U.S. who are transitioning through menopause, what you really want to know is why you can't find a comfortable pair of slacks without an elastic waistband. You may also wonder why your usual quick-fix method of knocking off a few pounds to fit into a dress no longer works or why all your extra fat is accumulating around your middle.

Welcome to Mid-life! An Equal Opportunity Event

This is a time of enormous change. Whatever you call it, the pause, the passage, perimenopause or menopause, this change affects your body, your mind and your spirit. But, don't despair; there really is a good reason for all these changes.

Change is good. It knocks you out of your complacency. The enormous changes you are experiencing right now are an opportunity to view your body and your weight in an entirely different light. Without the burden of having to strive for that perfect body, you can now focus on a healthy body. So throw out the scale and give up the notion of perfection.

Consider this irony: The changes in your body—the wider waist, the extra fat around your middle, the discarding of the belt—represent perfection at its finest. Your body is working perfectly, doing exactly what it was designed to do at this time in your life.

But before I reveal the physiology behind the perfection, let me assure you that I truly understand your desire for a healthy body. I know you want to live a long and healthy life, a life free of chronic disease. I bet you are also concerned about heart disease, osteoporosis and breast cancer and that you want to remain active with energy to participate in all that life has to offer. I know too, that many of you have dreams of watching your grandchildren graduate from college and start lives of their own. Or maybe you have dreams of traveling, starting a new business, writing a book, ending world hunger or finding a cure for AIDS. Or maybe your dream is of living in a peaceful world, one that is free of terrorism and violent crime.

How do I know this? Because hundreds of women just like you have told me so in the classes I teach and in my practice. I know that your heart is in the right place, but you are distracted by all the changes that are taking place in your body. You want answers *now*, so you can take control of the battle of the bulge before you succumb to a one-size-fits-all wardrobe.

Weight Control Throughout Menopause

Again, your body is an amazing creation. It knows what you need to thrive through all its physical changes. You not only survived puberty, you went on to blossom beyond puberty. That was a time of extreme change. As your hormones kicked in you developed breasts, hips, pubic hair, menstrual periods and mood swings. Then, during pregnancy (if you've been pregnant), your hormones kicked in again, propelling your body through another round of changes: your breasts grew, your tummy expanded, your hips widened, your feet grew sometimes a whole shoe size, and just when you didn't think your tummy could get any bigger, it grew some more.

Now, during menopause, your body is changing again.

And, yes, it is because of hormones. This time you have hot flashes, night sweats, mood swings, decrease libido, vaginal dryness and sleep disturbances because you don't have enough hormones. So, why is your waist expanding? Why is the scale telling you that you have gained ten pounds?

Mid-life weight gain, believe it or not, happens for many sound physiological reasons. Try to stop cursing your waistline for a minute while we explore the reason your body is taking on extra fat cells at this time in your life.

Body Fat Relieves Menopausal Symptoms

As you age you lose muscle mass. From the age of 35 on, the average woman loses about a half a pound of muscle per year. At the same time she gains—or replaces that muscle—with one and a half pounds of fat. Muscle burns fat. Muscle also speeds up your metabolism. When you lose muscle you lose your ability to burn calories. The more muscle you lose, the fewer calories your body needs. The more sedentary (non-physically active) you are, the more muscle mass you lose. And suddenly you're caught up in a vicious, negative cycle.

Your body, in its infinite wisdom, knows that as you transition through menopause your ovaries and adrenal glands dramatically reduce their production of estrogen. Your body also knows—even if you don't—that you still need a certain amount of estrogen to:

- keep your hot flashes at bay
- keep your skin moist
- keep your heart and bones healthy
- keep your brain functioning and,
- support about 295 other systems in your body to allow you to live a long and healthy life.

And, your body has some pretty creative ways of producing enough estrogen to support these functions.

Fat Cells With a Job to Do

Estrogen can be produced by your fat cells. The larger the fat cell, the more estrogen it can produce. Your body does this by producing more fat-storing enzymes and fewer fat-releasing enzymes. This mechanism kicks in as the estrogen production from your ovaries and adrenal glands slows down with age. Studies have shown that women with the largest fat cells produce 40 percent more estrogen than women with the smallest ones. In most cases women going into menopause with more fat on their bodies have an easier transition with fewer symptoms than women who are thinner.

The location of the fat is important as well. Abdominal fat cells are more conducive to producing estrogen. Abdominal fat cells surrounding the liver and adrenal glands help produce estrogen through the enzyme releasing and conversion process. The adrenal glands also produce testosterone, which is converted into estrogen by an enzyme that the liver produces. So there you have it. Your body knows how to protect you and keep you more comfortable through the menopause transition by increasing the amount of fat stored in your fat cells, which in turn provides what's called endogenous (from within) estrogen. Once again, your body does what it needs to do in the best way it knows how. The body doesn't take into consideration culture-based beliefs such as "thin is better" nor does it worry about how your clothes fit or how it appears in a mirror. Your body's sole purpose is to keep you alive and comfortable through these major physical transitions.

By now you are probably thinking, *Great, I'm glad my*

Feelin' Hot?

body knows what to do to see me through these changes, but I still want to lose this extra weight.

Details, Details. It's Always About the Details

The answer, of course, is in the details.

- The details of paying attention to not only how much you eat, but what you eat.
- The details of moving your body through some form of regular aerobic exercise and strength training.
- The details of changing your attitude from "How can I be thinner?" to "How can I be healthier?"
- The details of reordering your priorities from fitting into a size six dress to living the rest of your life free from disease and disability.

Let's start with calories. The first step involves a balancing act. You need to start balancing your intake of calories with how many calories you burn each day. At the same time, instead of focusing on your weight, focus on how much muscle mass you are building and how much fat you are losing. The only way this will happen is with consistent aerobic and strength-training exercise.

This balancing act contains no magic. It is not the current fad diet. It is not a diet at all. If you're like most women, you have tried several magic diets in your time and experienced some initial success. But the weight returns a few months later after you went off the magic diet. Picture your metabolism as a furnace that burns calories. By building more muscle mass through consistent exercise your metabolism will burn more calories and burn them efficiently. Your goal is to improve your overall health, not to get your 22-inch waist back. If you need guidance and support with your eating habits, Weight Watchers is an excellent program.

The Right Kind of Diet

Make sure your calories come from foods that feed and nourish your body. I'm talking about fruits and vegetables, and especially plant-based proteins such as bean, lentils, legumes and soy. Soy is an excellent example of a plant-based protein. Many studies support soy's ability to lower cholesterol levels, ease hot flashes, and keep your heart strong. And if you're not big on tofu, don't worry; it's not the only source of soy. You can buy soybeans, soy nuts, soy milk and soy cheese, all of which can be easily integrated into your meals. What makes soy foods so beneficial? Soy contains isoflavones (a natural plant compound), which produce estrogen-like effects in the body, which in turn help protect you from heart disease and improves your overall health.

Eat More But Less

You will gain better control of your eating by balancing meal portion size with meal frequency. Studies have shown that you burn more calories when you eat five small, frequent meals each day, rather than three large ones. Why is this so? Every time you eat the digestion process begins and this process requires energy, which in turn revs up your metabolism. A faster metabolism burns more calories. Eating more frequently also stabilizes your blood sugar level. Without wide fluctuations in blood sugar, you will be less hungry at each small meal. A drop in blood sugar triggers not only hunger, but also symptoms like shaking, fatigue, mood swings, and an inability to concentrate. You may already be dealing with fatigue, inability to concentrate and mood swings due to menopause so why add to your symptoms? You need stability, not more chaos.

By eating five small, frequent meals and keeping your blood sugar stable you will not eat in excess. This eating method will give you more control over the calories you consume and the ones you burn. In no time at all, you will feel the difference in the way your clothes fit. Remember it's not how much you "weigh" it's how good you feel.

A Healthy Body Requires Exercise

Now the time has come to talk about exercise. You didn't think I was going to forget to mention exercise, did you? You may be thinking, *I've tried exercising,* or *I don't have time to exercise.* Or *I don't like to exercise, it's not fun.* If you feel this way, it's OK. I'm still going to talk about the importance of daily exercise in your life.

Remember, I promised to tell you the truth about menopause? Well, here's the truth: To live a long and healthy life beyond menopause, one that is free from disease and disability, you must exercise! Before you start any exercise program, of course, you should check with your doctor. If weight loss is your goal, you will probably need to exercise at least four times a week for thirty-minute periods. If you don't have 30 minutes at one time, studies have shown that you can derive the same benefits by exercising ten minutes, three times daily. Once you are fit and weight loss is no longer an issue, you can maintain your fitness level with exercise just three days a week.

Exercise has many, many benefits. It:

- Improves your mood
- Helps you sleep better
- Builds muscle mass,
- Reduces stress
- Burns calories
- Makes your clothes fit better

Need I say more?

I am sure you have read about ways to incorporate exercise in your daily life, such as taking the stairs instead of the elevator or parking your car further away from the building. Actually, this is a good way of remembering where you parked your car at the mall. Your car is always the one parked alone in the furthest corner of the parking lot. These are good suggestions, ones that I hope you are already using. But, if you need more support in putting exercise on your priority list and keeping it there, here is an idea.

Find a cause that you feel passionate about such as multiple sclerosis, AIDS, muscular dystrophy, breast cancer or heart disease, and become involved. Societies exist for each of these diseases, and they all need help raising money. Every year these societies host a walk, run, hike, bicycle ride or swim in every major city across the U.S. By training for one of these events you will be doing two important things: exercising your body and raising money for a wonderful cause.

Several years ago, Avon hosted a three-day walk all over the country to raise money for breast cancer. My best friend and I trained for and completed Avon's first three-day walk. We had to raise a certain amount of money just to be able to participate in the walk. Avon provided training groups and tips to prepare us to successfully complete the three-day walk. We trained for almost nine months before the event. Studies have shown that it takes about six weeks to change any behavior. So, by committing yourself to one of these causes and participating actively, you can change your behavior from sedentary to active. The physical benefits you receive during this process will encourage you to keep up a regular exercise program as an important part of your daily life.

You will also meet some amazing people. The Avon event I participated in is now called the "Breast Cancer 3-Day." The National Philanthropic Trust Project now sponsors it and 85 percent of the net proceeds from the 3-Day benefit the Susan G. Komen Breast Cancer Foundation. You can find more information regarding this 3-day walk online at www.breastcancer3day.org. Check newspapers, libraries and women's magazines for information about other fund-raising activities. Keep your eyes open; there are many causes that need your support.

If you enjoy walking and being outside, you may also enjoy hiking. The Sierra Club plans hikes almost every day of the week in cities large and small all over the U.S. and in many international locations as well. Hiking will help you burn calories while maintaining strong bones and a healthy heart. Hiking also feeds your soul with the intrinsic beauty of nature. You can hike at your own pace and still receive all the same benefits listed above.

Exercise: Where Do I Find The Time?

If you are like most women I talk with, time is an issue in your busy life. I hear this concern every time I discuss the need to include exercise as part of a healthy lifestyle. If time is holding you back, I highly recommend the books and philosophy of a woman named Cheryl Richardson. Cheryl is the author of several books including: *Take Time for Your Life,*

Life Makeovers and her most recent book, *Stand Up for Your Life*. As a personal coach and author, Cheryl will open your eyes to new ways of thinking about how you spend your time.

Although making exercise a daily priority was not an issue for me, believing that I could make my dreams come true certainly was. By following the suggestions in Cheryl's books, attending her life-enhancing retreats, and reading her inspiring newsletters each week, I am using my time more wisely, and effectively to make my life the very best it can be. I know that you can, too. Sometimes all you need is the right support. You can find out more about Cheryl's programs by visiting her website at www.cherylrichardson.com. Her books are available at all major bookstores, the library, and on the web at Amazon.com.

So now that you know that time is of the essence and weight is not the issue, let's move on to finding out how to keep your heart beating strong all the days of your life.

Feelin' Hot?

Chapter 8

Let's Get to the Heart of the Matter

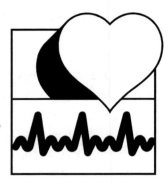

In the absence of wake-up calls, many of us never really confront the critical issues of life.
— Unknown

When I think of the word "heart," I seldom think of my physical heart. I think, instead, of the color red or a heart-shaped valentine or feelings of love. Not until I reached the age of menopause did the word "heart" make me think about the physical heart that beats in my chest.

How often do you think about the health of your physical heart? Do you take for granted its seemingly inexhaustible work ethic or do you wonder if it's properly conditioned to continue the job? If you are like most of us, you never question your heart's physical state until it sends out a warning symptom or two.

Heart Disease – The Number One Killer

Hopefully, your heart hasn't sent out any warnings yet. If all is well, it is in good working order with no physical complaints and will remain so. But the absence of warning symptoms is no reason to be complacent about your heart's heath. Statistics about the development of heart disease in women over the age of 50 are staggering.

Did you know that one out of every two women over the age of 50 will die from heart disease? Most women don't. They are far too worried about the specter of breast cancer to think much about their hearts. While public awareness regarding breast health has undoubtedly saved lives, the sad fact is that heart disease will kill more women than breast cancer, uterine cancer and ovarian cancer combined.

So, now you know the truth, and with knowledge comes power; the power to make the necessary lifestyle changes to beat the statistics. In the past most heart disease research and prevention efforts were focused on the male population, but now researchers are spending just as much time, energy and money on the prevention of heart disease in women.

So why does heart disease become a major health risk for women after menopause? Why don't women start developing heart disease earlier, as many men do? And why is it that women often do not survive their first heart attack? The answers to these questions are vital to our survival.

As it turns out, one of the wonderful hormones produced by our ovaries, adrenal glands and fat tissue ever since we went through puberty is the same one that protects our hearts from disease. And that hormone is—you guessed it— estrogen. At least, estrogen protected your heart prior to menopause.

Estrogen — The Great Heart Protector

If you have read this far, you are aware of the importance of estrogen to your health. Your heart also depends on estrogen; at least it did when estrogen was available. Behind the scenes estrogen has been keeping the vessels leading to the heart dilated, protecting them from narrowing, hardening and generally becoming constricted. It has also helped stop the development of plaque while keeping your cholesterol levels and blood pressure within normal ranges.

Unfortunately, with the onset of menopause and the subsequent reduction in estrogen production, you begin to lose vital protection. If you don't have healthy lifestyle habits in place, like sensible eating and regular exercise, your arteries may start to harden. Plaque can develop at an alarming rate, and your arteries may start to narrow. This paralyzing process will reduce the flow of oxygenated blood to your heart. And when your heart no longer has an adequate blood supply, it will make its problems known!

So, if estrogen is so important to our hearts and vessels, why don't we just take some estrogen and be on our way? Because ongoing clinical trials do not support this hypothesis. The Women's Health Initiative Study results, which were published in July 2002, showed an *increase* in heart attacks and strokes in women who were taking a combination of estrogen and progestin. Other studies done prior to the Women's Health Initiative also support these findings.

Getting That Heart Checked

Heart attack and stroke are the two life-robbing effects of untreated and undiagnosed heart disease. Several tests are available to help determine if you're at risk for developing heart disease. If you haven't had a complete physical in the last year, then you should schedule one with your primary care physician soon. When you arrive at your appointment the doctor will most likely want to do the following:

- Listen to your heart and lungs, and take your blood pressure. Your blood pressure is an important indicator of general health or potential problems. The guidelines for healthy blood pressure are changing. They are much stricter than they once were. In the past 130/85 was somewhat reassuring. Now cardiologists are suggesting 120/80 as a healthier number to shoot for.

- Obtain a fasting cholesterol panel. The results give your doctor additional information regarding your overall risk of heart disease. There are five essential components to the cholesterol panel, all of which your doctor should discuss with you when the results come in.

  1. Total cholesterol should be less than 200.
  2. Triglycerides. This is the scientific name for calorie-packed fat. Cardiovascular experts now know that at high levels, this fat can trigger a heart attack or stroke even if your cholesterol levels are normal. High triglycerides are an indication (especially for women) that heart disease may be developing. 150 or less is the number to shoot for.
  3. HDL. This is the good cholesterol that helps prevent plaque from forming in the arteries. Ideally, this number should be greater than 45. The higher the number the more protection there is against heart disease. The best way to increase HDL cholesterol is regular exercise.
  4. LDL. This is considered the "bad" cholesterol. Ideally the number should be 130 or below.

Feelin' Hot?

5. HDL/Cholesterol ratio. Divide your total cholesterol by your HDL cholesterol. If the resulting number is 4 or less you are at low risk for heart disease.

- Check your weight. Your weight and where you carry it is a risk factor for heart disease. If you carry most of your extra weight around your waist, you are said to have an apple shape. An apple shape can put you at risk for diabetes, which in turn can increase your risk of heart disease.

- Check your blood sugar. When your blood is drawn for the fasting cholesterol panel, a fasting blood sugar level is also tested from the same sample. If your fasting blood sugar level is normal, no further testing is needed for diabetes at this time. If the test level is not normal, then further tests may be required.

My Mission: Improving Every Woman's Life

The prevention of heart disease is always preferable to the treatment of heart disease. Strange as it may seem, simply recognizing a heart attack in women has become a vital concern for the medical community. Many women have died having their first heart attack because the classic symptoms men experience—such as crushing chest pain that radiates down the left arm—is not always present in women. Heart attacks in women have many times been mistaken by the medical community as anxiety and treated inappropriately. For this reason women are more likely to die of their first heart attack than men. Women who are entering menopause today are fortunate in the amount of information, encouragement and support available to help them prevent heart disease. Our mothers and grandmothers weren't so lucky. This point became very obvious to me over the Thanksgiving holiday last year when my mother-in-law came to visit.

The day after Thanksgiving the two of us went shopping. Of course, I picked the busiest shopping day of the year to hit the mall. Unlike many women, my shopping gene—if I have one at all—is extremely recessive. So, to break up the day we stopped at a restaurant for lunch and—wouldn't you know it—so did everyone else in the mall. While we waited to be seated, people came into the restaurant in droves.

As I sat there, I was saddened that most of the people who were around my parents' age did not appear to be healthy. I overheard a gentleman discussing his recent quadruple bypass surgery. This major surgery is performed on people who have damaged arteries due to heart disease. A woman who sat down next to me showed visible signs of having suffered a stroke; her speech was slow and somewhat slurred. I started talking with the woman's daughter who told me how grateful she was that her mother was able to join her on this shopping spree after the months of rehabilitation that followed the stroke. Many other people came into the restaurant that day using wheel chairs, walkers and canes. What I found so discouraging was that these people were in their 70s, not their 90s. At that moment I vowed to educate as many women as possible on healthy ways to avoid these situations. My mission now is to help women improve the quality of their lives.

Information Is Everywhere

We baby boomers have been fortunate in the messages

we grew up with in regards to our health. Our parents' generation smoked heavily and did not relate to the concept of exercise. Many of us never smoked, or did so for only a short time. On the downside, we grew up in the grab-a-burger-and-run generation. That's because us female boomers have been in the work force most of our adult lives, and have been raising families at the same time. We are left with little time or energy to exercise. And meal planning is a matter of getting our families fed and off to the next activity. Our do-it-all lifestyle has fostered some unhealthy habits that we now must honestly evaluate and change.

For a while the medical community gave us the erroneous message that if we took hormones, particularly estrogen, we would most likely avoid heart disease without exercise or healthy eating habits. Now, thanks to the many women who participated in the Women's Health Initiative clinical trial, we know that this is not true. While estrogen provides many protective benefits before menopause, it does not appear to have the same protective benefits after menopause.

So... how do you prevent heart disease without the magic hormone pill? Read on...

Lifestyle choices will always be your best hedge against heart disease and other chronic illnesses. Awareness that heart disease is the number one killer of women over the age of 50 is a good place to start. Another important step is to acknowledge that you have some control over preventing this disease and then accept responsibility for it. An honest assessment of your nutrition and exercise habits is a must.

Diet: A Key Player

The diet that is most effective against heart disease (and

I'm sure you have heard this before) is one that is:

- low in saturated fat
- high in fiber
- rich in nutrients

No more grabbing a burger at a fast food chain. I am talking about a diet that is loaded with fruits and vegetables as well as plant-based (rather than animal-based) proteins. It should also include omega three fatty acids (such as those found in certain fish, including salmon, mackerel and canned tuna) at least three times a week. The medical community has expressed concern recently about high levels of mercury found in fresh tuna from the store or in sushi. At this time, it is probably best to limit your intake of fresh tuna.

Soy is an excellent source of plant-based protein. As I have already said, soy can come from soy milk, soy beans, soy nuts, and tofu. Many cereals have now added soy protein. If you are having bothersome hot flashes, adding soy to your diet may help ease them. It is better to get your soy protein from food sources rather than supplements.

High-quality snack bars can provide soy and other nutrients. One of my favorite sources of soy protein is the Luna Bar, which is made by Clif Bar Inc. The Luna Bar is a whole nutrition bar made especially for women. My daughter introduced me to it when I was visiting her in Chicago. We had just finished a long day of shopping (Oh God). I was starving, but I didn't want to spoil my appetite for dinner. So my daughter gave me a Luna Bar. Wow! From that moment on I was in love with the Luna Bar. Why? Well, it tastes delicious, comes in a variety of different flavors, and is packed with nutrients that every woman's body needs. The one I ate that day is called *Nutz Over Chocolate*. Need I say more? Most importantly though, the Luna Bar has 8 to 9 grams of soy protein, 23 vitamins and minerals, including a full day's supply of folic acid, and 350mg of the 1500mg of calcium that we need each day. And of course, we know the importance of adequate amounts of calcium in our diet to protect our bones.

Folic acid is an important mineral to include in our diet each day as well. Studies have shown that folic acid helps to reduce a form of inflammation called homocysteine that can be present in our blood. High levels of homocysteine have been found in men and women with heart disease. The Luna Bar is also wheat and dairy free. This is important to many women who have developed sensitivities to these substances as they've aged. And just when you think it can't get any better, the Luna Bar has only 180 calories and 4 grams of fat. Although I was *Nutz Over Chocolate* in Chicago, my favorite flavor now is *Peanut Butter 'n Jelly.*

Clif Bar Inc. actually donates a portion of the money you spend on Luna Bars to the Breast Cancer Fund, which really touches my heart. You can find more information about the Luna bar in the resource section located at the back of this book.

Oh No...the Exercise Word Again!

It is finally time to discuss the importance of exercise in the prevention of heart disease. You didn't think I was going to skip exercise, did you?

Daily exercise is one of the best protectors against heart disease. While certain kinds of exercise are more protective of the heart than others, every form of exercise is beneficial. I realize that many women don't feel they have adequate time to exercise, nor do they have the desire to add exercise to their already enormously long to-do list. I also know that your health care practitioner doesn't always have the time during your very short visits together to drive home the importance of exercise to your long-term health and longevity.

That's why I'm doing it here.

The kind of exercise that best protects your heart is aerobic exercise, which is any activity that increases your heart rate, requiring you to use more oxygen. Aerobic literally means "with oxygen." Many studies have shown that women who use more oxygen through aerobic activity can reduce the risk of premature death from heart disease by *300 percent*. Aerobic exercise can help lower blood pressure, increase the good HDL cholesterol and reduce the bad LDL cholesterol. In addition, aerobic exercise enlarges the arteries to the heart and improves blood flow to this amazing muscle.

You can achieve an aerobic benefit from just about any exercise that you enjoy. Whether it is walking briskly, hiking, jogging, dancing, skiing, tennis or even bowling, golfing or swimming, any of these will help. Finding the time to do these activities becomes another challenge.

Finding the Time

I find that if I do my walking, hiking, or jogging first thing in the morning, my whole day goes more smoothly. I use this time to work out problems in my mind. It is similar to meditation, but I don't have to sit still. By allowing my mind to wander, so to speak, I don't think about how much further I have to go. Before I know it, I have come to the end of my walk or hike, and I am ready to tackle the day. I advise walking with a friend. It helps pass the time, and the commitment helps both of you stick with the program.

Walking or hiking in the early evening during spring and

summer months is a nice way to end the day. My local branch of The Sierra Club sponsors late afternoon/early evening hikes at least once a week in addition to their weekend hikes. The Sierra Club is a wonderful organization that arranges hikes for all levels of fitness. You will meet wonderful like-minded people who will support your efforts to improve your health.

Speaking of hiking, I know you have the desire to keep your heart healthy. And now you have the awareness that heart disease is the number one killer of women. So, take out your do-to list and write, "Keep my heart healthy" at the top, and make sure it stays there.

Being Responsible to Your Health

Your continued day-to-day quality of life depends on the decisions you make regarding your health. In the past your responsibilities to your family and work may have hindered your decision to include healthy eating and regular aerobic exercise in your daily regimen. By now, you realize that the responsibility you have to yourself is just as important as the responsibility you have for your family.

In the next chapter I will talk about another part of your body that needs special care after menopause: your bones! You probably don't think about your bones very often because, like your heart, they are hidden from sight. But, without strong bones, the mobility you have always taken for granted will begin to slip away.

The good news is that the steps you take to keep your heart healthy will also keep your bones healthy. Let's move on so I can encourage you to develop a healthy relationship with your bones.

Chapter 9

No Bones About It

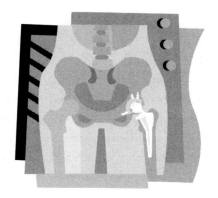

Protecting your body from disease and disability becomes extremely important during and after the menopause years. After decades of focusing your energy on the care of other people's health, it's time for you to devote the same energy to your own well-being.

When the physical symptoms of menopause scream for your attention, it's easy to know where to focus your energy. Once you do, you will quickly know whether your efforts have paid off; the symptoms either subside or they don't. But your bones, like your heart, are hidden from sight, and seldom show any sign of damage until the damage is done. But never forget that the strength and integrity of your bones are vitally important to your overall health.

How Solid Is Your Frame?

Have you ever watched a construction crew frame a house? It's a simple concept, I know, but without a solid framework the house will not be able to support the weight and stress of its load. No matter how much money is spent on the walls, paint, fixtures or furniture, the house won't survive the test of time without a healthy, strong framework.

When I was a child of seven, I prayed that I would break my arm. Can you imagine that? But I was a child, and I saw that when other kids broke their arms they got to wear a cast and sling, which brought them an enviable amount of attention. Well, I wanted that attention for myself. So I made a cardboard cast, painted it white and taped it together so it would stay on my arm. I finished off the look by making a sling out of one of my father's old shirts.

This episode in my life had two fortunate outcomes. First, my make-believe cast and sling satisfied my immature desire to have a broken arm. Eventually I lost interest in the guise and moved on to other fantasies. The second fortunate outcome is that I matured without actually breaking an arm or resorting to other potentially dangerous ploys for attention.

Many years later in a high school anatomy class, I watched the teacher trying to bring the skeletal system to life. All I saw was the skeleton of a very dead person hanging from a hook. I set about the business of memorizing the names of the bones so I could pass the test and get a good grade in the class, but for some reason I just couldn't relate to the significance of the skeletal system. It wasn't until I was in nursing school that I finally realized why I was blocked. I had been looking at the skeletal system as a hard, dry, inactive, and a very dead homework assignment.

Our Bones Are Alive

Alive, but out of sight, over 200 bones are hard at work not only framing your body, but also protecting your vital organs, like your brain, heart, lungs, kidney and liver. Your bones also contain a huge repository of essential minerals, especially calcium. Minerals are vital to the proper functioning of many organs in your body. We all know that calcium builds strong bones. But did you know that many vitamins such as C, D, and K are also essential for strong bones? The bottom line is that without a strong skeleton system your body would lack the support it needs not only to stand upright and move from place to place, but to lend support to the organs through its repository of vitamins and minerals.

Is Your Bone Crew Asleep At The Job?

Every bone in your body has its own blood and nerve supply as well as its own cellular network. This system works night and day to maintain the strength and integrity of your skeletal system. If you could get a peek at your bones under a microscope, you would see what looks like a very large construction site manned by busy bone cell crews. One crew is responsible for demolishing old bone, while another crew quickly comes by to rebuild with new bone. This is called remodeling, and the health of your bones depends on this very complex process. The crews of cells that demolish and replace bone have special names. Osteoclast cells clear away the old bone material and osteoblast cells rebuild the bone with new material.

Remodeling and replacing old bone with new is a complex activity. Inside your bones this process takes place automatically and continuously, similar to the beating of your heart, seemingly without your input or control. I say seemingly because the truth is you do have some control over how well your bones are working. In fact, the condition your bones are in at mid-life is a reflection of your eating and lifestyle habits going back to when you were a child, a teen and a young adult.

But don't let that deter you. Fortunately, it is never too late to start a healthy bone building and protecting routine. By including a variety of foods, possible vitamin and mineral supplements, as well as several forms of exercise, you can not only maintain and preserve your bones you can improve their quality as well. I will introduce this bone-building routine to you a little later in this chapter. For now, let's talk about diet.

What food comes to mind when you think of your bones? Perhaps you remember a slogan that was popular when you were a child: "To build strong bones and teeth you need to drink...your milk!" But, while milk is a good source of calcium (as are all dairy products); it is not the only way to build and protect your bones. I enjoyed drinking milk until I was a young adult. As a teenager I loved to come home from school and drink ice-cold milk right out of the carton, a habit that did not go unnoticed by my mother who repeatedly told me to pour it into a glass. By the time I reached young adulthood, however, I was no longer interested in milk. I rejected it as fattening and decided to spend my calories on something more urgent...chocolate! There just has to be some calcium in chocolate...right?

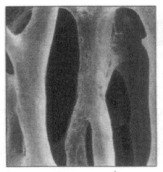
Normal Bone*

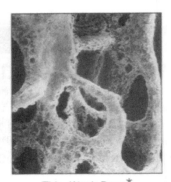
Thin, Weak Bone*

So, why all this talk about the skeletal system and the process of demolishing and rebuilding bone? You already know that healthy bones frame and protect your body, keep you upright and allow you to move freely. What you may not know is that this process of rebuilding old bone with new bone slows down when you reach the age of 35, at which point you may actually lose approximately one percent of your bone mass each year. Then, when you reach menopause and ovulation stops, the process of bone-mass loss may actually start to accelerate because of hormone reduction. The loss of too much bone mass can lead to a condition called osteoporosis, which literally means "porous bone." The medical community defines osteoporosis as a chronic, progressive disease characterized by low bone mass. Because the bones can become very fragile, this condition puts you at risk of fracturing bones in your wrist, hip, or vertebrae (spine).

If you have the following risk factors, you may be predisposed toward osteoporosis:

- Female gender (of course)
- Advanced age
- Caucasian or Asian race
- Family history of osteoporosis
- Small and/or thin boned
- Physically inactive lifestyle
- Lack of adequate calcium and vitamin D intake
- Use of certain prescription medications such as steroids, and anti-seizure drugs.

Thyroid disease with excessive doses of thyroid medication and premature menopause can be added to this long list, too. Whew! With a list like this, it's amazing we have any bone mass left by the time we reach mid-life.

Menopause and Accelerated Bone Loss

Osteoporosis has been called the silent disease because often there are no early warning signs. Studies have shown that when a woman goes through menopause she can actually lose anywhere from one to five percent of her bone mass per year. The average loss is around two percent. Bone density that is abnormally low, but not low enough to be classified as osteoporosis, is defined as osteopenia. Fortunately, osteopenia does not have to lead to osteoporosis. Education about these conditions and early detection is the key.

Determining Your Bone Density

How can osteopenia be detected early? The best way to determine the strength, integrity, density and total mass of your bones is the Dual energy X-ray absorptiometry scan, commonly known as the DEXA scan. The DEXA scan precisely measures the total bone density in the body, as well as the density of individual bones in the hip, spine, and arm. This simple, painless test involves lying down on your back

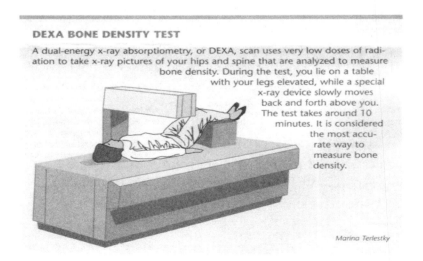

DEXA BONE DENSITY TEST

A dual-energy x-ray absorptiometry, or DEXA, scan uses very low doses of radiation to take x-ray pictures of your hips and spine that are analyzed to measure bone density. During the test, you lie on a table with your legs elevated, while a special x-ray device slowly moves back and forth above you. The test takes around 10 minutes. It is considered the most accurate way to measure bone density.

Marina Terlestky

and resting your legs comfortably over a cushioned pillow (see caption). Now how bad can that be? If the test wasn't so quick, you might be able to enjoy a short nap.

The x-ray used for the DEXA scan has only ten percent of the radiation in a chest x-ray. Until recently, you couldn't get this test unless you met certain criteria such as a family history of osteoporosis, a fractured bone, or being at least 65 years of age. Now, you can request this test as early as age 50. I advise all my patients to have their first DEXA scan at age 50. Why wait until you are 65 to find out that you have significant bone loss? The medical community has finally realized that to prevent osteoporosis from developing, bone loss has to be monitored as soon as it begins.

Understanding the Cause of Bone Loss

Let's talk first about the causes of bone loss, and then I'll explain measures you can take to avoid or minimize it. Even with a healthy lifestyle, some women may be genetically predisposed toward osteopenia or osteoporosis.

Before menopause your bones are protected by three major factors.

1. Hormones, especially estrogen, the sex hormone
2. Your nutritional habits
3. Regular exercise, particularly weight bearing activities such as walking, jogging, hiking or stair climbing, helps to determine the density and strength of your bone mass. Actually stressing a bone with weight (your weight) strengthens bone. Continuing a weight-bearing exercise program after menopause is a must. Adding

strength training to your exercise routine will give you added benefit.

In almost every chapter I have dealt with the major role hormones play in keeping your body running smoothly and helping you be the awesome woman you are. By now you appreciate just how special your sex hormones are to your body's overall health. Let's now explore how estrogen helps you maintain strong bones.

Estrogen (the goddess of all hormones) is primarily known as a sex hormone. Most women don't realize how vital estrogen is to the health of their bones. Your bones have special receptor sites for estrogen. Throughout your life bone mass has been rising and falling along with your estrogen levels. Estrogen is the hormone that is responsible for stimulating the bone-building activity of the osteoblasts. What's equally important is that estrogen is also responsible for suppressing the bone-dissolving activity of the osteoclasts. Before menopause the sequence of bone clearing and bone building was balanced by the production of estrogen. After menopause when your estrogen levels fall, the bone clearing operation speeds up and the bone building operation slows down. This delicate balancing act has become lopsided.

Estrogen also promotes the work of calcium and vitamin D in bone formation. Before menopause, estrogen helped your intestines absorb calcium from the foods you ate, while at the same time promoting conservation of calcium by the kidneys, which resulted in less calcium being excreted. But the Goddess Estrogen doesn't stop there. She also stimulates the activity of vitamin D, which is essential for calcium metabolism as well as indirectly regulating the release of many other hormones that affect the bones, including calcitonin, parathyroid hormone, growth hormone and last but never least, that male tag-a-long…testosterone.

As you can see, the menopause transition affects your physical being profoundly. It goes way beyond the cessation of your menstrual cycles and your ability to have children.

Are Men Susceptible to Bone Loss?

At this point, you may be asking yourself if men are susceptible to osteopenia and osteoporosis, too. The answer is yes. It has been estimated that approximately two million men have osteoporosis. But, the emphasis on early detection and treatment has been almost exclusively focused on women, leaving men, tragically, on their own.

Until recently, the medical community thought that because men have 25 percent more bone mass than women to begin with; they have natural protection against developing osteoporosis. This increased bone mass is due to the male sex hormone testosterone, which helps stimulate bone and muscle growth. Men produce approximately seven times more testosterone each day than women do. Whew! That's a lot of sexual thoughts. No wonder they don't have time to clean the toilet. Men also tend to be more physically active than women, and that activity helps build muscle.

As we learned earlier in this chapter, nutrition and diet help protect bone. Men typically are larger, more muscular and more active. To maintain their stature, they need to eat more than women do. With larger portions of food come more nutrients, especially calcium, which can be utilized by the body. Women can begin to have fractures due to osteoporosis as early as age 50, while men, thanks to a higher peak bone mass and slower bone loss, usually have another decade or two before they reach a critical point.

Before we got sidetracked discussing men (as we women

often do), I mentioned three factors that have protected your bones prior to menopause. The first was the hormone estrogen, which we just discussed. The second is your nutritional status. Good nutrition has and always will be an important player in maintaining your day-to-day quality of life. As you age good nutrition will continue to add to your longevity of life. What role does good nutrition play with keeping your bones healthy and strong?

The Healthy Lifestyle

A healthy diet that includes plenty of fruits and vegetables will provide most of the nutrients your body needs for good bone health. The two most important nutrients are calcium and vitamin D. However, ongoing research tells us that many other vitamins and minerals must be included in a healthy diet as well. Minerals such as magnesium, potassium, zinc, sodium and phosphorus are also considered important because our skeleton is formed from minerals. In fact, approximately 17 percent of our bone mass is derived from the mineral phosphorus. Vitamins C and K, as I mentioned earlier, are also important to good bone health. They both contribute in different ways to collagen production, which is the first stage of bone formation.

Vitamin Supplements

Now we know that good nutrition is essential in providing the vitamins and minerals necessary for strong bones. Unfortunately, research has also shown that most women are not eating foods that have enough of these vitamins and minerals. Therefore, it may become necessary to rely on supplements to provide the necessary nutrients for our bones. One drawback to relying on supplements is that we have to remember to take them! Most of us don't have a problem remembering to eat!

The most important supplement is calcium, with vitamin D and magnesium. You will need approximately 1500mg (milligrams) of calcium a day, including whatever calcium you are getting from your diet. If you eat 500mg a day of calcium, you need to make up for the remaining 1000mg with supplements. Remember to divide the calcium into two separate doses of no more than 500mg each to assure that your body will utilize all the calcium you take. Studies have shown that the body cannot absorb more than 500mg at one time. Also, check the label of the bottle to find the amount of "elemental" calcium in each tablet. Elemental simply means the actual amount of calcium contained in a compound. The less "elemental" calcium in each tablet, the more tablets you will need to take.

Vitamin D and magnesium help the bone absorb the calcium. You will need approximately 320mg of magnesium a day and 400 international units of vitamin D. If you eat lots of fruits and vegetables and get approximately 10 minutes per day of sun exposure, you are already getting all the magnesium and vitamin D you need, which means you can take a calcium supplement without vitamin D and magnesium. Some doctors advise their patients to take one of their calcium supplements at night before they go to bed. It's believed that you experience a mild increase in bone turnover during sleep that may lead to bone loss, compared with when you're up and moving around.

There are many different forms of calcium available, all of which can be purchased over the counter without a prescription. The two best forms of calcium are in calcium carbonate and calcium citrate. As I said above, the more elemental calcium in the tablet, the less calcium you will need. Calcium carbonate generally has more elemental calcium per tablet than calcium citrate. However, calcium carbonate needs to be taken on a full stomach because it requires stomach acid for proper absorption to take place. Calcium citrate, on the other hand, may be taken between meals. Calcium citrate generally has less elemental calcium per tablet; therefore you need more tablets to achieve the same dosage.

To summarize, all women should take calcium supplementation after menopause. For proper absorption, each tablet should have no more than 500mg of elemental calcium. The total recommended dosage is approximately 1500mg per day and any calcium-rich foods you eat each day count towards that dosage. One final word of encouragement: some research in progress suggests that a daily calcium intake of at least 1500mg may help burn fat!

Here Comes That Exercise Word Again

Earlier in this chapter I mentioned a bone-building routine to help maintain the strength of your bones. This routine will also help your body continue to build "new" strong bone throughout the rest of your life. So, what form does this routine take?

Two kinds of exercise that build and maintain strong bone are:

- Weight-bearing exercise
- Strength-training exercise

Remember, stressing the bone actually helps stimulate

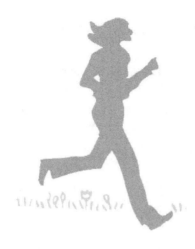

new bone growth. Weight-bearing exercises include walking, jogging, hiking, stair climbing, and tennis. Some researchers suggest that certain forms of yoga might also contribute to bone strength. Remember, as we age our muscle will be replaced with fat if we don't exercise.

Strength training is important as well and should be added to the routine. Use light weights, no more than 5 pounds. In many cases 2 or 3 pounds will do. The area to focus on is your upper body. By building strength in your upper body, you will increase the bone strength in your spine. An added benefit is stronger arms and leaner muscles. To achieve the best results, perform your routine three times a week. I recommend that you find a class that teaches good body mechanics and proper form. These classes are usually offered at a reasonable price at your local YMCA, community center or gym. An excellent book that provides all the scientific research, plus suggested exercises with pictures is: *Strong Women, Strong Bones* by Miriam E. Nelson, Ph.D. If you prefer to exercise to a video, I recommend *Moving through Menopause* by Kathy Smith.

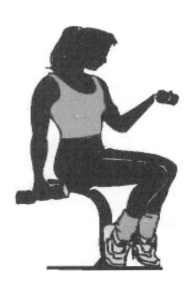

Feelin' Hot?

Can Hormones Keep My Bones Strong?

Many women ask "Should I take hormones, particularly estrogen, to maintain strong bones?" For many years now the medical community has recommended that all women take estrogen after menopause to protect their bones. As you know from previous chapters, there are certain risks associated with taking estrogen long term.

So what's a woman to do? My recommendation, which I'm sure you can guess at this point, is to first discuss your individual situation with your doctor. If you are at a high risk for breast cancer, a medication called Evista has been FDA approved for osteoporosis protection. Evista is considered a "designer estrogen" because it doesn't stimulate breast tissue, but does protect bones. The drawback is that it can cause more hot flashes. Once again, there is no perfect pill for everyone. No matter what you decide about estrogen therapy, remember that the bone-building routine that I described earlier with calcium supplementation and good nutrition is your best bet for a lifetime of healthy bones.

This chapter would not be complete without acknowledging that some women— despite their best efforts—may need to take medication not discussed in this chapter due to a diagnosis of osteopenia or osteoporosis. Whatever weight bearing and strength training exercises you do will further enhance the protection that this medication provides.

And finally, the last chapter of this book is just ahead. In case you haven't already peeked, this chapter introduces my systematic approach to making decisions regarding menopause easy, with minimal stress. I will introduce to you the SHOP method. Most women love to shop, but no woman likes to be sold. Read on to find out how you can become your best advocate for a long and healthy life.

Chapter 10

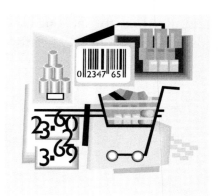

What's a Woman to Do?

The quickest way to know a woman is to go shopping with her.
— Marcelene Cox

One of my goals when I sat down to write this book was to provide women with an easy, intuitive means of making critical lifestyle choices during and beyond menopause. I have developed a fun, methodical approach, which we will explore together in this final chapter.

First, let's review the journey we've taken together so far. By now, you've acquired an understanding of the common menopause symptoms and their causes. You've also developed an appreciation for the delicate balancing act that takes place within your body, mind and spirit during this wonderful, but difficult stage of life.

And, as you've heard me say over and over, the single defining message of this book is: "Many women, many choices." It was erroneous for us members of the medical profession to ever think otherwise. The many women who have stood up to the notion of "one size fits all" have been courageous in saying enough is enough. I've described each menopause symptom in detail. But, for each symptom, rather than telling you how to treat it, I have suggested many treatment options, from conventional hormone replacement therapy to homeopathic cures and aromatherapy. I know that each of you will find your stride as you explore your options.

So, again, what is a woman to do? How do you decide which of the many approaches is best suited to you as an individual? How do you discover what areas of your unique health history you should focus on first? Who should you consult when you have questions regarding your health?

A Methodical Approach

I am very excited to introduce to you a revolutionary new method called SHOP. I designed it with **you,** the woman, in mind. Once you start using the SHOP method your calmness will show, making your friends want to know all about it as well.

Now, you may be wondering how I, a woman whose shopping gene is admittedly recessive, could possibly know where to SHOP. When it comes to shopping for answers to health questions during and beyond menopause...well, I'm the expert. And just because I need a personal shopper to choose clothes for me, doesn't mean I don't know menopause like the back of my hand. I do. And I know the perfect place to take you for the ultimate menopause shopping experience.

Let's SHOP

Every woman enjoys shopping for something. I have little patience for clothes shopping but I can spend hours at a nursery choosing flowers for my garden. My best friend, on the other hand, can spend the whole day shopping for antiques.

But no matter what you, as a woman, like to shop for; you don't like to feel that you were <u>SOLD</u>!

Being sold means coming home with a product or service that doesn't feel right for you. This can happen regardless of what you are shopping for: a car, clothes, skin care products, and a health care service; it doesn't matter.

When you SHOP according to my method, you are in control. When you are SOLD, you feel like you were on the wrong side of a one-sided sale. I am going to show you how to be in partnership with your health care decisions without being sold on products or services you don't feel good about.

There are many ways to approach shopping, and every woman has her own unique style. By answering the questions below you will discover your style. Then I will show you how to apply that style to making health care decisions during menopause. So hold on ladies, we are going shopping!

Where are we going to shop? It's called Menopause Land. Dress in layers because the temperature can be fine one minute and then, without warning, it's hot, hot, hot. Wear comfortable shoes and a hat to shelter you from the sun. And don't forget your glasses because you'll want to see clearly. You won't be alone because the population of Menopause Land is 470 million women strong and growing fast. With so many women in residence you just know the shopping opportunities will be incredible. So...get ready for an incredible shopping trip to the highest peaks of Menopause Land. Once there, the view will give you a completely new perspective!

On Toward Menopause Land

Your passport to Menopause Land must be stamped with your shopping style, which we will determine in the quiz below. Then I will show you how to use your passport to make health decisions while living in Menopause Land. Let's first start by defining the acronym, SHOP.

S.H.O.P

Select a
Health care provider who is
Open to your
Point of view

Finding the right health care provider is the first decision you have to make, and it will impact all your subsequent decisions. Now, let's explore your feelings about menopause. Which of the two following statements best reflects your point of view?

- Menopause is a natural transition with physical symptoms that are temporarily inconvenient. This, too, shall pass.
- Menopause is a medical emergency that requires intervention by a medical specialist, followed by medication.

I have to assume it is the latter, otherwise you probably wouldn't be reading this book! Either way you will still need a health care provider with whom you feel comfortable.

Shopping Style Quiz

Check a. or b. in the following question sets about shopping for clothes.

1. a. _____ I find shopping a pleasurable activity.
   b. _____ I consider shopping a chore.
2. a. _____ I choose clothes off the rack myself.
   b. _____ I like to have a clerk choose clothes for me.
3. a. _____ I shop only out of necessity.
   b. _____ I shop regularly because I love to choose clothes.
4. a. _____ I always write an organized shopping list.
   b. _____ I am spontaneous and buy whatever catches my eye.
5. a. _____ I'm a trendsetter.
   b. _____ I prefer to wear what others are wearing.
6 a. _____ I like to browse for bargains and sales.
   b. _____ I pay full price so I can have first choice.
7. a. _____ I like to mix and match clothes.
   b. _____ I buy the whole outfit right off the manikin.
8. a. _____ I prefer to shop at large department and outlet stores.
   b. _____ I prefer a smaller, more unique selection at a one-of-a-kind boutique.
9. a. _____ I buy fully accessorized outfits with jewelry, shoes and bag.
   b. _____ I buy a basic outfit and defer accessorizing for later.
10. a. _____ When I buy something that doesn't fit, I put it away and never wear it.
    b. _____ I return it for something I can wear.
11. a. _____ I buy clothes for the parts of my body I like, while avoiding clothes for the parts I don't like.
    b. _____ I buy clothes for every part of my body whether I like it or not.

Now that you have a better idea of your unique shopping style, let's apply it to making health decisions. My goal is to make sure that every dollar you spend provides you with improved health, quality of life and longevity.

Question 1. You may need to shop around to find a health care provider who is open to your point of view. If you find shopping a pleasurable activity, you won't mind investigating the choices available under your particular health insurance plan. But if you find shopping a chore, you may feel a little anxious having to do the necessary footwork to find the best provider. If you recognize this up front, the anxiety will be reduced.

Question 2. The second question probes the amount of control you like to have over your health care decisions and the degree of interaction you like to have with your physician. If you want to have a controlling interest in your health care decisions, you will want to work with the kind of physician who will present a variety of options and then stand back and allow you to choose the one that is most appropriate to your style. But if you'd rather have your physician make the decisions, you will want to work with one who does not require your input. Most health plans allow you a choice of physicians. Make sure you have chosen the one who best suits your style.

Question 3. If you shop out of necessity, it's my guess that you only go to the doctor when something is bothering you. If so, I suggest that during your menopause transition you plan to visit your provider on a regular, scheduled basis (at least once a year). You may need more frequent visits in the early stages of menopause, depending on how you feel. On the other hand, if you shop regularly because you love choices, you are probably already in the habit of scheduling routine gynecology visits every year. This is an excellent habit.

Question 4. Before you go to the doctor, do you make a list of concerns or questions you want to discuss? Or do you wait and see what the doctor has to say? I suggest that when it comes to menopausal symptoms and controversial issues like hormone replacement therapy that you make a list to bring along. This way all your concerns will be addressed in a "designer" visit, rather than a knock off or generic version.

Question 5. If you are a trendsetter, you will probably be curious about alternatives or perhaps bio-identical compounding hormones. If you feel more comfortable doing what the majority of women are doing, conventional hormone replacement therapy may be your choice. Can you see the beauty of discovering your styles? There is no right or wrong choice here. Your style, preference and beliefs will generally ensure a successful outcome.

Question 6. If you like to shop for bargains and sales, generic prescriptive medications may suit you just fine. But if you spend the extra money for designer clothes, you will probably want to stick to a name-brand medication.

Questions 7. If you like to mix and match clothes from different manufacturers, you may want to try conventional medicine and complementary approaches together. For example, you might choose to complement hormone replacement therapy with aromatherapy. The mix and match approach makes it easy to incorporate a variety of health care methods together for an optimal outcome, which may be necessary for women who are dealing with myriad menopausal symptoms.

Question 8. Do you shop at large department and outlet stores or is a small, quaint, unique boutique more your style? If you are a boutique shopper, you will probably want to find a health care specialist such as a gynecologist who specializes in menopause or a woman's health nurse practitioner and menopause clinician like myself. On the other hand, if you prefer one-stop shopping, a family practice doctor with a nurse practitioner might be more your style

Question 9. When shopping for clothes do you focus on the whole, fully accessorized look or do you buy basics and add accessories as you find them? If you are a whole-look buyer, you probably want a comprehensive plan of care. You may be interested in hormone replacement therapy but you want to know how taking hormones will affect your bones and organs. You are also interested in how to approach exercise, vitamin supplementation, and diet at this time of your life. On the other hand, if you stick to the basics when shopping, your priority when visiting your provider may be symptom relief. You can consider the rest later.

Question 10. If you are willing to return an item that doesn't fit, you probably feel comfortable discussing the successes and failure of your health plan with your provider. If you are disappointed with the results you have experienced so far, but are reluctant to tell your doctor, perhaps you do not feel comfortable interacting with your health care provider. Many women think they are bothering their doctor if they call too often. <u>This is not true</u>. Your provider needs to know when something is not working for you. I will give you suggestions on how to make calls to your doctor a more positive experience.

Question 11. This last question may have been an "ah-ha" moment for you. Do you buy clothes for one part of your body while excluding the rest? If so, you are not alone. Most women favor certain parts of their bodies over others. But when it comes to your overall health and longevity, it's important to be inclusive of your whole body. If you religiously schedule a pap smear every year but have

Feelin' Hot?

mammograms only sporadically, you are leaving yourself vulnerable to a very serious health risk. Likewise, it's not uncommon for women to seek relief from the immediate physical symptoms of menopause while ignoring the less visible, but far more critical issues of their heart and bones.

Completing the SHOPping List

Now, let's put the whole package together. We're going to use the acronym SHOP again with a slightly different twist to help you focus on important issues when visiting your health care provider.

- **S**chedule an appointment with your **H**ealth care provider to discuss your **O**ptions for developing your **P**ersonal health profile.
- **S**elect the symptoms of your unique **H**istory and **O**rganize them in a list form, **P**rioritizing them from most to least bothersome.
- **S**pecial emphasis should be placed on screening you for **H**eart disease, diabetes, thyroid dysfunction, breast cancer, colon cancer, and **O**steoporosis, the results of which will be placed in your **P**ersonal health profile. Make sure your health care provider discusses the results with you.
- **S**ystematically focus first on the areas of your **H**ealth profile that needs immediate attention. **O**dds are we all have one area that needs our **P**ersonal attention.

- **S**hift your thinking from **H**oping you will retain your health as you age to knowing that you have **O**ptions. Then become **P**roactive in making sound decisions about your health.

I mentioned earlier that although all women love to shop for something, no woman likes to be **SOLD**. If this happens to you when visiting with your health care provider, you may feel like your confidence is **S**haken. They have given you very few **O**ptions, your doctor is not **L**istening to you and you have been left out of the **D**ecision making process. To turn this around into a **SHOP**ping experience, you should **S**top, take a deep breath and ask for **H**elp in exploring other **O**ptions; putting the **P**ower back where it belongs, with you.

Also remember, if the plan that you and your provider have agreed upon is not working, (the results you were hoping for are not forthcoming), the plan can always be changed!

You must let your doctor know when the plan or some part of it is not working. Yes, calling the doctor back can be intimidating, but you are the consumer and it's perfectly acceptable for you to call with questions or concerns. Jot down a few notes first to organize your thoughts. If your doctor communicates by e-mail—as many do these days—start the dialog via e-mail, which has the built-in advantage of forcing you to clarify your thoughts by putting them into words.

Few journeys through life are uninterrupted. Take these pauses as a time to reflect, refresh and recharge and they cease to be perceived as interruptions.

The Key to Life

It's Time To Go

The time has come for me to leave you here in Menopause Land. But I'm not really leaving; I have lived here for quite a few years. I sincerely hope that I have given you a positive look at this wonderful stage of life. Always remember that you are not alone. We are 470 million strong. Remember too, that while each of us is a unique individual, collectively we have far more similarities than differences. United, we have the power to make our future the healthiest that it can possibly be.

My final advice: Keep exploring your options and asking the hard questions. But also make time for your dreams, for it is in our dreams of the future where the hope of all mankind really lives.

And when in doubt, go shopping!

Bibliography for Further Reading

Ahlgrimm, Marla RPH and J Kells; *The HRT Solution: Optimizing Your Hormone Potential.* New York, NY: Avery Publishing Group, 1999

Burr, Ginger; *Fashion Secrets Mother Never Taught You.* Somerville Ma: Total Image Consultants: To order Toll Free 1-800-380-8726. On line orders: http://www.totalimageconsultants.com

Conrad, Christine; A *Woman's Guide to Natural Hormones: For Every Stage * For Every Age.* New York, NY: The Berkley Publishing Group, 2000

Cooke, John P., M.D., Ph.D., and J Zimmer; *The Cardiovascular Cure: How to Strengthen Your Self-Defense Against Heart Attack and Stroke.* New York, NY: Random House Inc., 2002

Lottor, Elisa Ph.D, N.D., and N Bruning; *Female and Forgetful: A Six-Step Program to Help Restore Your Memory and Sharpen Your Mind.* New York, NY: Warner Books Inc. 2002

Love, Susan M.D.; *Dr. Susan Love's Hormone Book: Making Informed Choices About Menopause.* New York, NY: Random House, 1997

Nelson, Miriam E., Ph.D; *Strong Women, Strong Bones: Everything You Need to Know to Prevent, Treat, and Beat Osteoporosis.* New York, NY: G. P. Putnam's Sons, 2000

Feelin' Hot?

Northrupp, Christiane M.D.; *The Wisdom of Menopause: Creating Physical and Emotional Health and Healing During the Change.* New York, NY: Bantam Books, 2001

Richardson, Cheryl; *Take Time for Your Life: A Personal Coach's 7-Step Program for Creating the Life You Want.* New York, NY: Broadway Books, 1999

Taylor, Eldred M.D. and Ava Bell-Taylor, M.D.; *Are Your Hormones Making You Sick?: A Woman's Guide to Better Health Through Hormonal Balance.* Lithonia, GA: Physicians Natural Medicine, Inc., 2000

Waterhouse, Debra M.P.H., R.D.; *Outsmarting the Mid-life Fat Cell: Winning Weight Control Strategies For Women Over 35 to Stay Fit Through Menopause.* New York, NY: Hyperion, 1998

Resources

Compounded Pharmacy

For questions regarding compounded hormones I recommend:

Elaine Blieden, R.Ph.
Pharmacist
Bio-identical Hormone Replacement Consultant
Panorama Compounded Pharmacy
6744 Balboa Boulevard
Lake Balboa, California 91406
Toll free number (800) 247-9767
Phone (818) 988-7979
Fax (818) 787-7256
Website: www.uniquerx.com
E-mail: uniquerx@aol.com

To find a local compounded pharmacy near you contact:

Professional Compounded Centers of America
(PCCA)
Toll free number (800) 331-2498 or (281) 933-6948
Fax (800) 874-5760 or (281) 933-6627

Salivary Hormone Testing

Great Smokies Diagnostic Lab
63 Zillicon Street
Asheville, NC 28801

Feelin' Hot?

Toll free number (800) 522-4762 (for doctors) or
(888) 891-3061 (for consumers)

Aeron Life Cycles
1933 Davis Street, Suite 310
San Leandro, Ca. 94577
Toll free number (800) 631-7900

Aromatherapy

For more information regarding the many beneficial effects
of aromatherapy and SwissJust products contact:

Patricia L. Caminiti
swissjustnatural@aol.com
(805) 492-5870

Video Tape- Moving Through Menopause by Kathy Smith

This 90 minute workout routine covers all the important
areas that a woman transitioning through perimenopause/
menopause needs to do to keep her body healthy. Visit
Kathy Smith on line at www.kathysmith.com or
www.sonymusicvideo.com

Luna Bar

For more information about LUNA – the Whole Nutrition
Bar for Women, visit their website at www.lunabar.com

About the Author

Rebecca J. Hulem, The Menopause Expert, is a Certified Menopause Clinician, Registered Nurse, Registered Nurse Practitioner, and Certified Nurse Midwife

For over 25 years Rebecca Hulem has shared her knowledge and expertise in the field of women's health. As a Certified Menopause Clinician, she specializes in educating women to understand the symptoms and behavior of the perimenopause and menopause transition. Bringing a refreshing message, and imparting the latest medical research, Rebecca empowers women to make informed treatment choices, with special emphasis on lifestyle management including nutrition, exercise and stress reduction.

Rebecca Hulem's mission is to use her book as a platform to reverse the notion that menopause is a disease. "My message is to remind women that this is indeed a temporary transition, and a natural passage," she states. "I encourage women to respect the 'pause' by taking time to reflect on their lives, and to make lifestyle changes that promote a long and healthy second half."

In her work as The Menopause Expert, Rebecca's activities include speaking engagements, customized workshops and individual consultations to a client list comprised of organizations, the medical community, and patients in her private practice. Her book, "Feelin' Hot?" reveals the truth about menopause in a light, humorous and informative way. Visit www.pausitivepassage.com for more information about Rebecca and her work.

About RJH Communications

When it comes to women's health issues, and especially menopause, women are easily overwhelmed by the advice and opinions of well-meaning friends and representatives of the medical community. Understanding these difficulties, Rebecca Hulem founded RJH Communications with the goal of supporting women throughout the transition and helping them make the journey as easy and as meaningful as possible. Countless publications describe in detail the clinical aspects of mid-life health issues. Hulem distinguishes herself by the belief that women, in their great diversity, deserve to be educated in the broadest way possible, beginning with the conventional approach of the traditional medical community and following through to the alternative body-mind-spirit approach of holistic medicine…and, of course, everything in between.

Rebecca has developed a variety of specific programs to help women on their journeys through the menopause years, making the transition a Pausitive Passage instead of a complicated, confusing problem. Rebecca encourages women to pursue their quest for answers by visiting her website and emailing questions and concerns. Please visit her at:

www.pausitivepassage.com

Rebecca's goals for her website are two-fold. One is to keep you informed as to the latest research and clinical information in an accessible manner. The other is to create a community of women who are looking for a meaningful transition. Read their comments and suggestions on topics including health, sexuality and well-being. Post your own comments so that others can benefit from your wisdom and experience.

If you are interested in a professional consultation individually, in a group setting, or via teleclass e-mail Rebecca at rebecca@pausitivepassage.com. She would love to hear from you.

RJH Communications
5737 Kanan Road, #261
Agoura Hills, CA 91301-1601

Quick Order Form

Fax orders: (818) 991-3570. Send this form

Phone orders: Call (818) 889-2475. Have your credit card ready.

Email orders: rebecca@pausitivepassage.com

Postal orders: RJH Communications, Rebecca Hulem, 5737 Kanan Road #261, Agoura Hills, CA 91301-1601

Please send _____ copies of *"Feelin' Hot?"* to the address shown below.

Please send more FREE information on: (Circle all that apply)

     Speaking/Seminars ____   Teleclasses ____   Consulting ____

Name: _____

Address: _____

City:_____ State: _____ Zip:_____

Telephone: _____

Email address: _____

Sales tax: Please add 7.75% for products shipped to California addresses.
Shipping:
US: $4 for the first book and $2.00 for each additional copy.
International: $9 for the 1st book and $5 for each additional product (estimate).

Payment: ___Check   ____ Credit Card:
       Visa ___ MasterCard ___ Discover ____

Card Number: _____

Name on card:_____ Exp. Date: ___ /___